THE MENOPAUSE METABOLISM

FIX

THE OVER-40 WOMAN'S 4-WEEK PROGRAM
TO RECOVER YOUR STRONG, SEXY (AND SANE)
SELF IN 15 MINUTES A DAY

CARA METZ

FAIR WINDS

Quarto.com

© 2025 Quarto Publishing Group USA Inc.
Text © 2025 Cara Metz

First published in 2025 by Fair Winds Press,
an imprint of The Quarto Group, 100 Cummings
Center, Suite 265-D, Beverly, MA 01915, USA.
T (978) 282-9590, F (978) 283-2742

All rights reserved. No part of this book may be reproduced in any form without written permission of the copyright owners. All images in this book have been reproduced with the knowledge and prior consent of the artists concerned, and no responsibility is accepted by producer, publisher, or printer for any infringement of copyright or otherwise, arising from the contents of this publication. Every effort has been made to ensure that credits accurately comply with the information supplied. We apologize for any inaccuracies that may have occurred and will resolve inaccurate or missing information in a subsequent reprinting of the book.

Fair Winds Press titles are also available at discount for retail, wholesale, promotional, and bulk purchase. For details, contact the Special Sales Manager by email at specialsales@quarto.com or by mail at The Quarto Group, Attn: Special Sales Manager, 100 Cummings Center, Suite 265-D, Beverly, MA 01915, USA.

29 28 27 26 25   1 2 3 4 5

ISBN: 978-0-7603-8916-4

Digital edition published in 2025
eISBN: 978-0-7603-8917-1

Library of Congress Cataloging-in-Publication Data

Names: Metz, Cara (Fitness instructor) author.
Title: The menopause metabolism fix : the over-40 woman's 4-week program to recover your strong, sexy (and sane) self in 15 minutes a day / by Cara Metz.
Description: Beverly, MA : Fair Winds Press, [2024] | Includes index. |
Identifiers: LCCN 2024020004 (print) | LCCN 2024020005 (ebook) | ISBN 9780760389164 | ISBN 9780760389171 (ebook)
Subjects: LCSH: Women--Health and hygiene--Popular works. | Menopause--Popular works. | Self-care, Health--Popular works. | Metabolism--Popular works.
Classification: LCC RA778 .M489 2024 (print) | LCC RA778 (ebook) | DDC 613/.04244--dc23/eng/20240521
LC record available at https://lccn.loc.gov/2024020004
LC ebook record available at https://lccn.loc.gov/2024020005

Design and Page Layout: Kelley Galbreath
Photography: Hester Barnes Photography and Film

Printed in China

DISCLAIMER Please note that by participating in any exercise or exercise program, there is an inherent risk of physical injury. Should you choose to engage in this exercise or exercise program, you do so voluntarily, assuming all related risks and acknowledge that Cara Fitness and any affiliated individuals or entities bear no liability whatsoever.

The content provided within this program is solely for educational purposes and does not replace professional healthcare advice, treatment plans, or services. It is crucial to consult with a physician or healthcare provider before initiating this or any other exercise program to determine if it is right for your needs.

Furthermore, the reproduction or retransmission of any portion of the exercise programs or information provided by Cara Fitness is strictly prohibited without prior written consent.

The material presented in this book is not to be considered a replacement for any professional medical advice or treatment. If you are pregnant, suffer from any medical condition, or are undergoing treatment for health issues, professional medical consultation is advised before adopting any advice or engaging in the practices suggested in this book. Additionally, it is imperative that you refrain from listening to the accompanying meditations while driving. Neither the creators, contributors, nor any individuals associated with the development of this publication accept liability for any injuries or damages that may occur because of following the guidance, exercises, or therapeutic techniques contained herein.

This book is dedicated to my girls.

Contents

Introduction

Menopause is a pivotal moment in a woman's life, a journey from where you are now to where you want to be. Along the way, you'll discover new things about yourself, experience a multitude of emotions, and face challenges. The good news is that this journey will also reveal a new you, with strengths, perspective, and capabilities that will empower you to face the future with confidence.

My mission is to be your guide and help illuminate your path as you navigate this profound journey. First, let me ask you a few questions.

Do you often find yourself feeling the following sentiments?

- I've gained weight but I'm not eating or exercising differently from how I was before.

- I have no energy or motivation. I feel I've lost who I am.

- I can't remember the last time I had a full night of sleep.

- I just can't get rid of this extra layer of fat around my belly.

- I often lose my train of thought and struggle to remember the simplest things.

- I feel anxious, overwhelmed, and my confidence is at an all-time low.

As a menopause fitness trainer, I hear this all the time from my clients. I too felt this way not so long ago! After a while, I noticed that the stories, the emotions, and the feelings of helplessness were the same. As I worked with these women, a composite picture emerged—an everywoman that I call "Jane."

Let's Meet Jane

Lately, Jane does not feel like herself. She is tired, irritable, and always feels a touch under the weather even though she knows she doesn't have a cold or flu. Most days she would rather just crawl back into bed. But each day, life drags her out with its commitments of work, home, and family. So, she begrudgingly gets up, drinks a couple of cups of coffee, and pushes herself to function. She is constantly on edge, and she may bite your head off over the most inconsequential thing. However, she's actually sweet and kind with a heart of gold.

Lately, she plasters a smile on her face to fight off any concerned queries, such as "'Are you okay?" or "What's wrong?" because she knows that she can only answer "Nothing. I'm fine!" a few more times before she cracks.

Jane has always been the glue that holds her family together. She has two almost-grown-up boys. One is away at college and a constant concern. It often feels all-consuming. She really wishes that he could be "out of sight, out of mind," but she worries about how he is faring so far away from home.

Her youngest boy is still a teenager living at home. He's just learning to drive. He's always been a bit more adventurous and daring than his older brother. Once he has his license, will he be safe and drive responsibly? She hopes so. Still, anxiety about both of her boys' welfare often keeps her awake at night.

She has been married for almost twenty-five years to her childhood sweetheart. He's a wonderful man but sometimes she wants to put a pillow over his head in the middle of the night simply because he is snoring peacefully while she tosses and turns. Why isn't he as worried about her boys as she is?

In fact, they have a happy marriage. Jane loves him very much, but she struggles to admit that sex is now an issue. She knows that lately he feels neglected but doesn't quite know how to talk to him about it. The problem is it just hurts down there and her self-esteem or even feeling sexy completely disappears when she looks at her ever-expanding belly in the mirror. Where, exactly, is all the flab coming from?

Even though Jane isn't eating differently than before and still does her twice-a-week dance fitness class, the weight just keeps piling on. She's tried to remain disciplined and not overeat, but she can't stop thinking about food. It has become an obsession, so much so that she's even started dreaming about what she can and can't eat.

On top of that, the guilt around food is so intense that it feels like it's driving her crazy! If she's really honest with herself, late-night snacking is becoming a big problem, which only makes her feel worse. Her husband often tells her that she is still beautiful, but she doesn't believe him. She wishes he would just stop saying what he thinks is the right thing to say!

Unfortunately, at work, things are stressful too. After years clawing her way to the top of the ladder, she now manages a team of twenty people. She loves her job but lately struggles to focus, especially when she needs to do a presentation. Sometimes, her brain just doesn't seem to work the way it should. Some days even remembering her own name can be difficult.

That's not all. Lately, she's been having hot flashes. It's embarrassing when her face burns like a furnace and sweat runs like a tap from her armpits. The younger team members try to hide their giggles but that just makes her feel mortified. Even worse, she can guarantee that the hot flashes will always be on a day when she's been up half the night with night sweats. Having to change the sheets at 3 a.m. instead of sleeping in a pool of perspiration just makes it even more miserable.

Jane desperately needs time to herself, but her needs are always last on the list. Things have intensified now that her mother has been diagnosed with early onset dementia. Dealing with her own emotions, coming to terms with what the future may hold, and now comforting her mom and helping her come to terms with her diagnosis is truly heart-wrenching.

Not only does she need to make plans for her mom's future, but she also needs to prepare her dad for what's to come. It doesn't help that they live a two-hour car journey away.

Jane feels like she's drowning. She's being pulled in so many directions that she doesn't know who she is anymore. Jane wants to feel better about herself, but her weight is creeping up and that makes her feel worse. But her time is limited, so it's difficult to find time to exercise.

Maybe a new outfit would perk her up, but she just can't find anything new to wear that she likes. Jane knows that she should wear something besides yoga clothes or sweatpants once she gets home, but right now, she needs to feel comfortable more than anything else.

Things are not right. Jane knows that she needs to make changes, but how on earth can she manage a new exercise routine? Her plate is already full. Yet, she knows she needs to do something because feeling like this is unbearable.

Each day is more difficult than the last, and Jane knows that something needs to change. But it's difficult to prioritize herself when everyone in her life—her husband, her kids, her parents, and her employees—need her so much. Focusing on herself would be selfish, but she just can't continue to function this way anymore.

If she does decide to act, where does she start? She's not even sure what the problem is!

Right now, her best solution and the thing she looks forward to the most after an exhausting day at home and work is a very large glass (or two) of red wine every night and a plate of french fries. Depending on the day, she sometimes drinks three glasses, hoping that it will help her sleep through the night.

When she wakes up, *Groundhog Day* is about to start again!

Does any of this sound familiar?

Do you see yourself in Jane? Believe me, I understand. I can promise you that it doesn't need to be this way. You can feel good again!

I've Been in Your Shoes

Hello. My name is Cara Metz. I am a fifty-year-old, perimenopausal woman. I am also a fitness coach who specializes in helping women over forty navigate the journey from peri- to postmenopause.

However, to be honest, for a long time I was ignorant as to how menopause and perimenopause affect us. It wasn't until I was in the thick of it myself that I began to study it so that I could help myself and my clients.

The Change

Perimenopause is the span of years that lead up to menopause. On average, it lasts seven years but can be longer or shorter. It all depends on the individual, as we are all different. This is the time that women start to notice symptoms such as irregular menstrual cycles, weight gain, and changes in mood, sleep, and sex drive, among other things.

For all the fanfare that menopause receives, menopause is not a period of time.

Menopause is the day when you have not had a period for one whole year. After that day, you're postmenopausal.

Before I experienced perimenopause, all I knew about *the change* was that this was when women experienced hot flashes and other symptoms. Once *the change* happened, and a woman's reproductive years were over, it seemed like she was past her prime, and it was all downhill from there. It sounded like bad news to me both in terms of how I could expect to look and feel.

Figuring Out the Problem

Even though I was forty-six when I started experiencing some of the symptoms of perimenopause, I never related it to menopause. I actually had no idea what was going on with my body.

It wasn't until I began to believe that I had early onset dementia because I couldn't remember people's names, where I parked my car, my workout routines when I was teaching, or even my train of thought mid-conversation that I knew I needed help.

So, I reached out to my best friend, Christina, and confided in her. Not only was I concerned that something was seriously wrong with me, but my confidence was also now at an all-time low. I was afraid to put myself forward in social or work situations just in case I made a fool of myself.

But talking to my friend made everything okay! Christina is a few years older than me. She had already experienced the transition to menopause. When I confided in her and told her what I was experiencing, she said, "That's menopause. You are going through the exact same thing I did. You're not crazy. Your hormones are playing havoc with your mind. Stop stressing. It will get better. You just need to ride it out."

This got me thinking . . .

Did I really have to ride it out?

How long would this last? (And did I really just want to endure it?)

So, I decided to do some research on menopause, and I was so surprised at what I learned! Menopause was the reason that I was distressed by the following:

I had trouble sleeping.

I experienced mood swings.

My confidence was at an all-time low.

I now had an added layer of fat on my belly.

I felt overwhelmed and anxious, had constant headaches, itchy skin, low libido, fatigue . . . the list goes on and on! It was all because of *the change*!

Menopause 101

So many women have difficulty acknowledging or accepting the onset of menopause. This can be due to various reasons, including fear of aging, lack of information, societal stigmas, or personal beliefs.

I'd never before even had a hot flash or many of my other symptoms, so it never occurred to me that all the things I was feeling and experiencing could be due to my changing hormones.

All I had ever heard was that women got hot flashes and that was menopause. End of story! But that's not so.

Finding Solutions: Feeling Like Yourself Again

Now, five years later, armed with a wealth of knowledge and renewed energy, I'm here to help you. I understand how it feels because I've been there too. I'm still figuring this time in my life out, but I promise to share everything I've learned with you.

My aim for the next four weeks is to guide you in a no-nonsense, practical, easy-to-follow plan so that you can begin to feel like *you* again. I'll teach you simple and easy ways to feel better. There's nothing complicated to learn or do.

Let's face it, we just have too much else going on in our lives for overcomplication.

What I do works, and it's simple, straightforward, and easy to follow. You just need to trust the process.

The 4-Week, 15-Minute Plan: Why It Works

The question I'm asked all the time is, "How can a four-week program with only fifteen-minute workouts make a difference?" My answer to this is that consistency is the key to results, and fifteen-minute workouts make it easier to make it a habit. The 4-Week, 15-Minute Plan gives you all the tools you need for continued success throughout and beyond this plan.

If you can stick with my plan for four weeks, you'll build the habits you need to not only reduce your menopause symptoms but also to lose weight and feel sexy and confident in your own skin.

How many times have you enthusiastically started a restrictive diet with endless amounts of exercise only to throw the towel in around week three? Let's face it. You're a busy woman with many commitments, and finding time for *you* on a continual basis is tough. That's why doing short consistent workouts is effective—you can fit them in and around your life and the workout is over before you know it.

Best of all, I've constructed the workouts so that you utilize the fifteen minutes to the fullest, and the results are incredible.

I'm so passionate about this plan because not only has it transformed my life and reduced my menopause symptoms, but it has also done the same for the thousands of women I've had the honor to work with.

If you trust me and trust the process, I promise that you'll also reduce your menopause symptoms, lose weight, feel full of energy, and feel confident in your own skin!

Are you ready to do this?

Yes?

Good for you! Okay, buckle up ladies. I'm going to take you on the let's-kick-menopause's-butt ride!

How to Use This Book

The best way to use this book is to read chapters 1 through 7 in part 1 to learn about menopause, including the symptoms, symptom relief, blood sugar regulation, nutrition, exercise, and having the right mindset. Each chapter in this section ends with "Action Steps" so that you can begin to put the program into practice.

However, you can also begin your exercise routine in part 2 and/or the dietary changes in part 3 and refer to the chapters as needed. It's up to you. Either way, you'll have the information, resources, and guidance you need to be your best self during this important transitional time in your life.

There are numerous helpful sidebars in the book that provide information and inspiration.

These include the following:

- **Menopause 101:** Information about menopause that you need to know

- **How to . . . :** Strategies that will help you make progress in the 4-Week, 15-Minute Plan

- **Small Steps, Big Results:** Spotlight on the rewards from taking consistent action each day

- **Did You Know?:** Research, information, and resources for you

- **Client Success Story:** Clients who have benefited from the program

- **Cara's Favorite Way to . . . :** My strategies to manage menopausal symptoms

Safety First!

It's important to always make sure you warm up before your workout. If you have a medical condition, an injury, or are pregnant, please get clearance from your doctor before you begin a workout regimen.

When you're ready to begin your workouts, always make sure that you have enough clear space around you to move freely and that all of your equipment is in good working order. Remember, if at any time during a workout you feel light headed, becomevery short of breath, or feel pain, please stop immediately and get medical help if you need it.

PART
ONE

Understanding Menopause: Problems and Solutions

Menopause: Is Your Body Breaking Up with You?

In this chapter, we'll explore the ins and outs of a normal menstrual cycle to make sense of the shifts your body is experiencing as menopause begins. I've also created a **How Are You Feeling?** symptom quiz that will help you to assess where you are right now in your 4-Week, 15-Minute Plan journey and what you most need to focus on to improve your health and well-being. Gaining clarity on both of these important aspects of menopause will help you better navigate this new and often challenging phase of life.

Ready to Dive Deeper?

To truly understand the many facets of menopause, first we need to take a step back and revisit the menstrual cycle. Think back to the time in your life before menopause began to make its presence felt. Like most women, your monthly cycle probably had its own rhythm. Sure, it might not have been like clockwork every time, but there was a pattern. With menopause, everything now feels thrown off balance, which is exactly what happens.

The Menstrual Cycle: The Calm Before the Storm

First, let's look at the phases of the menstrual cycle.

Menopause 101

Menopause is a natural biological process marking the end of a woman's menstrual cycle, typically occurring in the late forties or early fifties. It's confirmed when a woman goes without menstruating for 12 consecutive months.

Understanding this will help you understand the changes you're experiencing in menopause.

The menstrual cycle is a complex interplay of hormones that prepares the female body for a potential pregnancy. It usually spans around 28 days, although it can range from 21 to 35 days in adults and from 21 to 45 days in young teenagers. The cycle can be broken down into several phases:

MENSTRUAL PHASE: DAYS 1–5
What happens: This is the phase during which the uterine lining (endometrium) is shed, resulting in menstrual bleeding.

Energy and mood: Many women experience fatigue; and others, mood swings, irritability, or sadness. This is partly due to the drop in progesterone and estrogen right before menstruation starts.

Hormonal activity: Estrogen and progesterone levels are low.

FOLLICULAR PHASE: DAYS 1–14
What happens: The pituitary gland releases follicle stimulating hormone (FSH), which stimulates the growth of several ovarian follicles. One follicle becomes dominant and prepares to release an egg.

Energy and mood: As estrogen levels rise toward the end of this phase, many women experience a boost in energy, mood, and libido.

Hormonal activity: Estrogen levels start to rise to prepare the uterus for a potential fertilized egg.

OVULATION DAY: DAY 14 IN A 28-DAY CYCLE
What happens: The dominant follicle releases its egg in response to a surge of luteinizing hormone (LH).

Energy and mood: The surge in LH can produce heightened libido, and the peak of estrogen can create a sense of contentment or increased energy for some women.

Hormonal activity: There's a peak in estrogen right before ovulation.

LUTEAL PHASE: DAYS 15–28
What happens: After releasing the egg, the dominant follicle transforms into the corpus luteum, which secretes progesterone.

Energy and mood: Progesterone has a calming, sometimes sedative effect. As a result, some women feel more tired or temperamental. If the egg isn't fertilized, estrogen and progesterone levels start to drop, and many women experience PMS (premenstrual syndrome) symptoms such as irritability, mood swings, bloating, and breast tenderness.

Hormonal activity: Progesterone dominates this phase. Estrogen is present but in lower amounts compared to the follicular phase.

How Estrogen and Progesterone Affect Your Energy and Mood
Estrogen is often called a "feel-good hormone" because it boosts serotonin and serotonin receptors in the brain. This neurotransmitter can also promote higher energy levels, elevate mood, and increase pain tolerance.

On the other hand, progesterone has a calming, sometimes sedative effect. While it's essential for maintaining the uterine lining for a fertilized egg, its increase during the luteal phase can lead to feelings of fatigue. It also plays a role in body temperature regulation, which can impact sleep quality.

That said, it's important to recognize that every individual experiences the menstrual cycle differently. Factors like stress, diet, exercise, and underlying health conditions can influence the intensity and nature of symptoms. Some women might have very pronounced energy and mood fluctuations, while others might not notice them as much.

The Phases of Menopause: The Storm
Menopause is a natural biological process that signifies the end of a woman's reproductive years. This is a sign posted by a series of hormonal shifts that bring a unique range of symptoms along with long-term biological changes. So, even though menopause is a

Did You Know?

Menopause, technically, is just one day—
it's the day that marks consecutive months
without a menstrual period.

distinct event, it's also a process that leads to the end of the reproductive years and beyond.

1 **Perimenopause:** This is the transitional phase to menopause, as the ovaries gradually produce less estrogen. It often starts in a woman's forties, but can begin in her thirties, and lasts from four to eight years, although this can vary from woman to woman.

2 **Menopause:** This phase marks the official end of a woman's menstrual period, defined by twelve consecutive months without a period.

3 **Postmenopause:** These are the years after menopause. During this phase, many of the symptoms experienced during perimenopause may lessen, but the risk of certain health issues, such as osteoporosis or cardiovascular disease, can increase. This is due to reduced estrogen levels, which help to build and maintain bone strength and heart health.

4 **Hormonal Changes:** Throughout this process, the ovaries produce less estrogen and progesterone. Decreases in both hormones trigger the end of ovulation and menstruation. At this point, the pituitary gland produces higher levels of FSH to try to stimulate the ovaries.

The rhythmic ups and downs of menstruation have now been replaced by the process of menopause, or what I like to call *the storm*. That's because hormones are decreasing and, in turn, fluctuating, which is why we experience a myriad of symptoms that can make us miserable.

This is why understanding the menstrual cycle and the phases of menopause is so important. We need to understand that we are *not* going crazy but rather experiencing a process: the end of the cycle of menstruation and the transition to menopause.

To help you gain clarity about what you're experiencing and to help you focus on the symptoms you need the most help with, I've created a menopause symptom quiz that will tailor your 4-Week, 15-Minute Plan just for you.

Action Steps

1 **Remember that understanding** what's happening to your body at this unique juncture, the process from menses to menopause, is the first step to finding solutions to your symptoms.

2 **Go slow.** Take some time to slowly digest the material so you don't experience an information overload.

3 **Take the quiz** so you know what symptoms you'd like to focus on in your 4-Week, 15-Minute Plan. This will enable you to find solutions so that you can feel better, faster. In the next chapter, we'll learn about the six most common menopausal symptoms.

Quiz:
How Are You Feeling?

I recommend taking the quiz now and taking it again after you've worked through the 4-Week, 15-Minute Plan. My clients are often surprised to discover how many feelings and experiences can be tied to menopause and how much the four-week plan helps to alleviate their symptoms.

Rate each symptom on a scale from 0 to 5, with 0 indicating no presence of the symptom and 5 signaling that it's highly problematic. In other words, it's impacting your day and your life. Try to set aside a quiet time when you won't be disturbed and assess how you really feel as you go through this list. Remember, there are no right or wrong answers; just do the best you can.

What Do You Experience?

- [ ] Hot flashes
- [ ] Insomnia
- [ ] Irregular periods
- [ ] Mood swings
- [ ] Night sweats
- [ ] Anxiety
- [ ] Overwhelm
- [ ] Weight gain
- [ ] Brain fog
- [ ] Memory lapses
- [ ] Low libido
- [ ] Fatigue
- [ ] Irritability
- [ ] Pins and needles
- [ ] Joint pain

- [ ] Muscle aches and pains
- [ ] Sore breasts
- [ ] Electric shock sensations
- [ ] Weak bladder
- [ ] Vaginal dryness
- [ ] Itchy skin
- [ ] Depression
- [ ] Headaches
- [ ] Burning mouth
- [ ] Cravings
- [ ] Heart palpitations
- [ ] Irritable bowel syndrome (IBS)

- [ ] Bloating
- [ ] Osteoporosis
- [ ] Increased allergies
- [ ] Urinary tract infections (UTIs)
- [ ] Difficulty concentrating
- [ ] Thinning hair
- [ ] Low confidence
- [ ] Increased urination
- [ ] Dizziness
- [ ] Brittle nails
- [ ] Change in taste
- [ ] Panic attacks
- [ ] Increased belly fat

2

The Top Six Menopausal Symptoms

How'd you do on the quiz?

Did you notice that several of your symptoms scored high?

Did more than half get a rating of at least 3 or above?

Or perhaps you had fewer symptoms, but they're still affecting how you feel?

Even if just one or two symptoms are making a major impact on your life, it's a sign that you need help and that the 4-Week, 15-Minute Plan can work for you. You can reduce your symptoms and feel better. I'm going to help you understand *why* all of this is happening and what you can do about it. So, stay with me.

When I first took the quiz, I was surprised by how many symptoms I had and how they were affecting my life. I thought that this kind of thing affected *other* women, but not me, and that I'd sail through menopause effortlessly. Oh, how wrong I was!

The clients that I work with also struggle with a range of symptoms, many of which you might find familiar. These include the following:

- **Hot flashes:** An unexpected rush of warmth, typically felt in the upper body

- **Night sweats:** Hot flashes during the night that interrupt sleep

- **Sleep disturbances:** When you're unable to sleep through the night and uninterrupted rest feels like a distant dream

- **Mood shifts:** Feeling like you're swaying on a constant mood swing, with bouts of sadness, anxiety, and irritation

- **Belly Fat:** Gaining weight around the waist even though your eating habits haven't changed

- **Vaginal symptoms:** As estrogen levels dwindle, this can lead to dryness, discomfort, and atrophy

- **Brain fog:** Moments of forgetfulness or when your brain feels like it's wrapped in cotton

- **Urinary issues:** Feeling the need to go more often or suddenly and being more prone to UTIs

- **Bone concerns:** A decrease in bone density, upping the risk of osteoporosis

- **Libido lows:** A lowering desire for intimacy

- **Anxiety spikes:** A newfound or intensified sense of worry about things that used to feel trivial

From this list, I've highlighted six of the most common symptoms experienced by my clients. These include belly fat, hot flashes, brain fog, anxiety, sleep challenges, and diminished libido. Recognizing them is the first step to understanding and addressing them.

Belly Fat

Menopause is a transformative time in a woman's life, and one of the most notable changes many of us witness is the shift in where our body stores fat. To understand this, we need to explore the complex hormonal dance that our bodies perform.

THE OVARIAN ESTROGEN ERA

Your ovaries have been producing estrogen for most of your life. Estrogen is key not only for reproductive functions, but it also determines where fat is stored in our bodies. When we're younger, it favors the hips and thighs. But as you transition to menopause, the production of estrogen from your ovaries begins to fluctuate wildly, eventually dwindling down to virtually nil. With this reduction in ovarian estrogen, your body's original game plan is disrupted.

THE ADRENAL BACKUP

Your body, being the resilient system that it is, has a backup plan. Enter the adrenal glands. These tiny powerhouses are two small, triangular-shaped glands located on top of each kidney. Their primary role is to produce and release certain hormones that your body needs, especially in response to stress. Think of them as our built-in "emergency response centers."

When they are not overburdened, they produce a subtler form of estrogen to partially fill the void left by your ovaries. Sounds great, right? But here's the catch: Your adrenal glands are also responsible for managing stress through the release of hormones like adrenaline and cortisol. In our often-hectic modern lives, frequent stress and erratic blood sugar levels mean your adrenal glands are constantly on high alert, pumping out these stress hormones. This leaves little room for them to produce the backup estrogen we need.

THE BELLY FAT SAFETY NET

Your body is all about survival and adaptation. When the primary and secondary sources of estrogen falter, your system brings in the reserves. Fat cells, especially those around the abdominal area, can produce estrogen too. So your body, in a bid to maintain some estrogen balance, starts storing more fat in the belly area. This isn't out of spite, although it may feel that way! It's actually a protective mechanism. The body thinks, "Hey, if these fat cells can help produce even a smidgen more estrogen, let's keep them around!"

The irony is that while your body is trying its best to regulate hormonal balance by deploying fat cells, when you look in the mirror, the dreaded belly fat makes you feel stressed. This emotional turmoil further engages your adrenal glands, creating a vicious cycle.

In essence, this is your body's intricate response to declining estrogen, a mix of evolutionary survival strategie, and modern-day stressors. What's the silver lining? With the right guidance, understanding, and lifestyle strategies, you can navigate these changes with confidence and poise. By understanding this complex dance of hormones and their

Client Success Story

I tried for years to reduce my belly fat to no avail. I tried the 4-Week, 15-Minute Plan and within a month, I could see a noticeable difference and did not feel so bloated. The program is simple and easy and gave me amazing results!

—JANICE

roles, you empower yourself to make informed choices, manage stress, and embrace this phase of life with all its nuances.

Hot Flashes

Hot flashes can be miserable. Why do they happen? It's all thanks to a tiny region in your brain known as the hypothalamus. Often referred to as the body's "thermostat," the hypothalamus regulates your core temperature by integrating information from the body and the external environment. Hot flashes happen because the hypothalamus is affected by the hormonal fluctuations that occur during menopause.

HORMONAL MAYHEM AND ITS EFFECTS ON THE HYPOTHALAMUS

As perimenopause progresses into menopause, estrogen levels begin to decline. Apart from its reproductive role, estrogen also plays a pivotal role in communicating with the hypothalamus. When estrogen levels decrease, the hypothalamus can misinterpret the body's core temperature as being too high, even if it isn't. This means our reliable thermostat starts receiving mixed, sometimes incorrect, signals.

THE BODY'S COUNTERACTION

When the hypothalamus perceives an increase in core temperature, even if it's just a false alarm, it initiates a rapid cooling process. Blood vessels close to the skin's surface dilate (known as vasodilation) to release heat. This results in that all-too-familiar sensation of sudden heat and redness. To counteract this, the hypothalamus activates our sweat glands, leading to perspiration, an efficient way to cool the body down.

THE UNPREDICTABLE NATURE OF HOT FLASHES

The exact timing and intensity of hot flashes can be as unpredictable as the hormonal fluctuations themselves. They can strike during the day or disrupt a peaceful night's sleep and result in night sweats. The experience varies from woman to woman. Some might feel a mild warmth, while others face intense heat episodes that drench them in sweat.

UNDERSTANDING TRIGGERS

While hormonal change is the catalyst, certain external factors can exacerbate hot flashes. Spicy

HOW TO . . . *Discover Your Triggers*

When you have a hot flash, keep a log of what you've eaten and how you feel. This can help you pinpoint certain triggers that may cause a hot flash. Awareness is key when trying to reduce symptoms. Knowing what may cause hot flashes is the first step to reducing them.

foods, caffeine, stress, and certain medications can stimulate the hypothalamus further, leading to more frequent or severe episodes.

Brain Fog

Hormonal fluctuations can also cause brain fog. This was my main symptom, and I thought I was going crazy. I decided to learn more about why brain fog occurs and what I could do to reduce my symptoms.

BRAIN FOG, HORMONES, AND MENOPAUSE: WHAT'S THE CONNECTION?

Our brain, the incredible organ responsible for your memory, emotions, decisions, and intellect, doesn't function in isolation. It's intricately linked to the dance of hormones within your body. As women journey through menopause, this dance sometimes feels more like a chaotic mosh pit, with brain fog often crashing the party.

Estrogen is the hormone most intricately intertwined with cognitive function. When levels fluctuate, the brain's access to this crucial energy source can be inconsistent, leading to moments of mental "power outages."

Normally, estrogen aids in regulating the brain's availability of glucose (its primary energy source), supports mitochondria (the powerhouses of our cells), and plays a significant role in neurotransmission (the transfer of information between the nerve cells).

Neurotransmitters, the chemical messengers that send signals from a nerve cell to another nerve cell, muscle cell, or gland, include serotonin, dopamine, and norepinephrine. They act as messengers to ensure that your neural networks are firing smoothly. Disrupted levels can result in miscommunications or delays in message transmission, much like a faulty phone line.

Small Steps, Big Results

Brain fog was one of my most bothersome menopause symptoms. Overhauling my nutrition really helped to make a difference. When I decided to focus on eating nutritious foods and reduce my consumption of processed food, it was a game changer for me. I immediately began to feel better.

Menopause can be a stressful period, both emotionally and physically, which can trigger the release of another important hormone known as cortisol. Elevated cortisol levels over prolonged periods can also impair cognitive function and memory. It's like fog that rolls in. You just don't see things as clearly, and this can be very frustrating and debilitating.

THE SLEEP CONNECTION

Sleep disturbance, a common result of menopause, further compounds the issue. The brain needs restful sleep to repair, detoxify, and consolidate memories. Poor sleep equals a groggy brain, which, when combined with hormonal fluctuations, just makes brain fog even worse.

Anxiety and Feeling Overwhelmed

Many women who have symptoms of anxiety or feel overwhelmed go to their doctor, only to be prescribed antidepressants. I've spoken to many women who've had this experience. If more health practitioners were knowledgeable about the symptoms of menopause, this wouldn't happen as frequently. There is a definite connection between menopause and emotional well-being. Learning about this link will help you to understand why you feel the way you do and empower you to do something about it.

Menopause and Emotional Turbulence: Navigating This Tricky Time

Menopause is a profound journey, both physically and emotionally. For some, the emotional ebbs and flows are just as significant, if not more so, than hot flashes or night sweats. If you suddenly find regular activities, like driving on the freeway, attending social events, or everyday tasks triggering anxiety, you're not alone.

HOW HORMONAL CHANGES AFFECT EMOTIONAL WELL-BEING

Two primary hormones—estrogen and progesterone—determine much of your emotional landscape during menopause. Estrogen is more than just a reproductive hormone; it's also intricately linked with serotonin, the brain's feel-good neurotransmitter. A decline in estrogen can mean a consistent drop in serotonin levels, making you more susceptible to mood swings, anxiety, and feelings of sadness.

Progesterone often acts as a mood stabilizer. As its levels taper off during menopause, the calming, mood-balancing effects can diminish, leading to heightened anxiety and emotional sensitivity.

CORTISOL MAKES SYMPTOMS WORSE

Life during menopause often involves dealing with other major life transitions such as adult children leaving home, career shifts, caring for aging parents, and confronting our own mortality as we

Menopause 101

If you're feeling emotionally exhausted, know that your experience is valid and shared by many other women. Remember, you are part of a vast community of women who are on the same journey, with similar challenges. Together, we can find strength and solace and know that we are, indeed, not alone.

age. These stressors, combined with the physical challenges of menopause, can elevate cortisol levels. Excessive cortisol can also exacerbate anxiety and the feeling of being overwrought, making emotional waves feel more like tsunamis.

Sleep Deprivation

As estrogen levels fluctuate, it can affect your sleep patterns too, which can lead to insomnia. This means that instead of getting a restful night's sleep, you may have to contend with night sweats, racing thoughts, and sleep deprivation. Navigating this temperature seesaw can feel like a desert one moment and freezing cold the next!

That's not all. Where once you could count on progesterone to help you fall asleep, diminishing levels of this hormone mean you'll be awake during the night instead of getting the rest you so desperately need. Hormonal shifts can also sometimes cause blood sugar spikes and subsequent crashes, which can lead to midnight hunger pangs. That silent call from the kitchen can disrupt your sleep patterns even further.

Low Libido

During menopause, many women experience a decrease in sexual desire. This shift can be due to both physiological and psychological factors. Often, women keep this symptom to themselves because they're embarrassed that they no longer have the desire for sex. This can lead to problems in relationships because partners suddenly feel rejected.

The good news is that there is something you can do about it. Understanding why your libido has gone AWOL can help you to find ways to solve this problem and to talk to your partner about it.

One of the primary causes of decreased libido during menopause is the drop in estrogen levels. Estrogen plays a pivotal role in maintaining vaginal health and lubrication, supporting sexual arousal, and contributing to mood stabilization. Progesterone, known to play a role in maintaining libido, also declines during menopause. Testosterone levels also decrease. While this hormone is usually associated with men, women also produce testosterone, albeit in smaller amounts. As women approach menopause, levels of this hormone decline, which impacts libido as well.

Did You Know?

Conversations about sexual health during menopause are not just necessary, they're a gateway to empowerment and satisfaction. When you address sexual issues openly and honestly, whether with your friends or partner, you're moving out of silence and isolation and toward understanding, support, and connection. Your story can also help others.

Vaginal Dryness

Lower estrogen levels also lead to vaginal dryness. As estrogen decreases, the tissues of the vaginal walls can become thinner, less elastic, and drier. This dryness can make intercourse painful, further contributing to a reduced interest in sexual activity.

Navigating menopause can feel like moving through a maze of unexpected changes, from sudden belly fat to hot flashes, from anxiety and feeling overwhelmed to brain fog, sleepless nights, and lost libido. But there is hope. In the next chapter, we'll explore each of these symptoms and more and provide Action Steps that will give you relief.

Action Steps

1 **Keep a log of the symptoms** you're experiencing. How does each symptom affect you? How often does it occur?

2 **Which symptom affects** your life the most right now?

3 **Decide which symptom** to focus on.

4 **Go to chapter 3** and read about the Action Steps to take with this symptom. If you have more than one, do one symptom at a time. Go slow. You don't have to do everything all at once.

3

Simple Solutions to the Top Six Symptoms and More

Now that you have a better idea of the symptoms that you'd like to focus on, whether it's belly fat, hot flashes, brain fog, anxiety and feeling overwhelmed, sleep deprivation, or a low libido, you'll find answers here. Practicing these tips and strategies over time will decrease your discomfort and help you feel better.

Later in the book, we'll add exercise and recipes to help you change how you move and eat. All the tools in the 4-Week, 15-Minute Plan work together to improve your outlook as you travel through menopause and beyond.

Reducing Belly Fat

1 Embrace a Balanced Diet: When it comes to belly fat, the most important thing you can do is to focus on fruits, vegetables, lean proteins, complex carbohydrates, and whole grains for a healthy plate. You need a wide range of nutritious whole foods so that your body has all the nutrients it needs to help lose that unwanted weight around the middle.

That's because the belly fat that shows up in menopause is visceral fat. It's not the same as subcutaneous fat that can build up all over the body. Subcutaneous fat is the soft, pinchable, fat that sits just beneath the skin. Think of it as the body's cushioning. Reducing this fat can often be achieved by maintaining a calorie deficit; that is, consuming fewer calories than we burn. Visceral fat is the more hidden type, tucked away deep around our abdominal organs. It's not just about aesthetics. High levels of visceral fat can also be a health concern.

Here's the catch: Simply cutting calories won't target this stubborn fat effectively. To combat visceral fat, the focus needs to shift from quantity to *quality*. It's about nourishing your body with nutrient-dense foods that support your hormonal balance and overall wellness. In essence, while a calorie deficit might help shed some pounds, it's the quality of our diet that plays a pivotal role in addressing the deeper, visceral fat, especially during the menopausal phase.

2 **Say "No" to Sugary Treats:** Too much sugar in your diet causes your blood sugar to spike, then crash. As the blood sugar crashes, the adrenal glands go into overdrive, producing adrenaline and cortisol to try and lift you up again. Unfortunately, there's lots of sugar in many of the foods that you eat, especially processed foods.

To reduce belly fat, begin by being mindful of what is *in* your food. Make it a habit to check the labels of the food you buy. Your best bet is to not eat food that comes prepackaged. It's not always easy, but if you can eliminate this type of food, you'll be on the right track.

3 **Incorporate Strength Training:** Use weights and resistance exercises to tone and firm your muscles and increase bone density. Add some form of strength training at least three times a week to your routine. Creating more lean muscle allows your body to work at rest, burning any unwanted calories.

4 **Cardio Workouts:** Engage in activities like brisk walking, dancing, or swimming. Do some form of movement that you enjoy each day, not just for a cardio workout but also for your mental health. If you feel better mentally and emotionally, you're far more likely to make better food choices. As a bonus, activity, rather than making you tired, will actually give you *more* energy and a zest for life!

5 **Lower Your Stress Levels:** Manage stress with relaxation techniques, like deep breathing and yoga. This gives your adrenal glands a break because it helps reduce the amount of adrenaline and cortisol that are produced, which can add to belly fat.

Remember, you can't always get rid of all the stress in your life, but you can decide how you'll react. Learning relaxation strategies may not

seem connected to belly fat, but stress relief does help reduce that extra weight around the middle.

6 **Prioritize Quality Sleep:** Aim for adequate sleep to support your weight management goals. This can be difficult because disturbed sleep will lower your reserves and willpower. This can lead to quick-fix poor food choices such as high-processed, high-sugar foods in an effort to lift your spirits and energy. Unfortunately, these foods can spike your blood sugar levels and lead to a crash.

Sleep disruption also impacts the balance between leptin and ghrelin, the hormones that regulate appetite. Leptin suppresses appetite, whereas ghrelin stimulates it. With poor sleep, leptin levels tend to decrease, and ghrelin levels increase, which can result in an increased appetite and potential overeating. Think of ghrelin as the hunger gremlin. We need to keep the little gremlin under control so that it doesn't disrupt your hunger hormones.

Furthermore, chronic sleep disruption can also slow down the metabolic rate. This means the body

CARA'S FAVORITE
WAY TO . . .

Get a Good Night's Sleep

Do your best to close the kitchen after 8 p.m. or at least three hours before bed. Snacking late at night can lead to sleep disruptions when your blood sugar spikes and then crashes, which causes adrenaline and cortisol to be released. You wake up and feel tired, but wired, and then are unable to fall back to sleep!

burns fewer calories at rest, which can lead to weight gain over time.

Dial Down the Heat of Hot Flashes

Hot flashes can be an uncomfortable rite of passage in your menopausal journey, but learning why they happen, specifically the role of the hypothalamus, can help you to take control. These tips and strategies will enable you to manage and even reduce their frequency and intensity.

1 Stay Cool and Hydrated: Wearing light clothing and drinking enough water (if your mouth is dry, drink) can help counteract sudden temperature spikes.

2 Try Mindful Breathing: Slow, measured breathing can calm the nervous system and reduce the intensity of a hot flash.

3 Choose the Right Foods: Phytoestrogens (plant-based compounds that mimic estrogen in the body) found in foods like soy and flaxseeds can help to reduce the severity and frequency of hot flashes.

4 Experiment with Herbal Remedies: Certain teas, like black cohost and red clover, can offer some relief.

5 Monitor Your Triggers: Keeping a detailed diary can help you identify specific triggers and help you to avoid them.

Navigating Brain Fog

Brain fog during menopause, while frustrating, is a natural result of hormonal changes taking place

Did You Know?

Cognitive behavioral therapy (CBT) provides practical, evidence-based methods that can help you navigate hot flashes and enable you to build resilience and remain composed and in control. These strategies can equip you with techniques that address not only the physical sensations that accompany hot flashes but also the emotional responses that may arise. Embracing CBT can be a significant step toward mitigating the intensity of hot flashes and help you reclaim a sense of comfort and confidence in daily life.

during this time. Learning strategies to enhance cognitive function can help you navigate this foggy phase of your life and move into a feeling of self-awareness and empowerment. Focus on these tips to keep your brain sharp and agile:

1 Feed Your Brain: Prioritizing a brain-boosting diet is key. Omega-3 fatty acids, antioxidants, and B vitamins play pivotal roles in cognitive health.

2 Regular Physical Activity: Exercise improves blood flow to the brain and supports neuron growth and neurotransmitter balance. It's also important when it comes to relieving other menopausal symptoms, which is why it's a key component of my 4-Week, 15-Minute Plan. You'll find more in part 3.

3 Mental Stimulation: Like your body, your brain benefits from a good workout. Regular reading, puzzles, and learning a new language or a new skill keeps the brain agile.

4 **Stress Management:** It's important to find ways to manage stress because it helps to keep cortisol in check. Yoga, meditation, and deep breathing exercises can all help you to relax.

5 **Sleep Hygiene:** Establish a regular sleep routine. Wake up and go to sleep at the same time each day. Make sure your bedroom is comfortable and the right temperature. Avoid stimulants like caffeine and alcohol close to bedtime. Don't watch or read the news right before bed.

Ease Anxiety and Stop Feeling Overwhelmed: Creating an Oasis of Calm

The emotional challenges of menopause can feel daunting. Understanding the hormonal changes behind these feelings can offer empowerment. Equipped with knowledge, you can actively seek strategies to nourish your emotional health.

1 **Dietary Harmony:** Consuming a balanced diet with mood-stabilizing foods, like magnesium-rich leafy greens, complex carbohydrates, and omega-3 fatty acids, can support emotional equilibrium. Including foods such as spinach, whole grains, and fish like salmon in your diet helps regulate mood swings and reduces stress levels. This is because the nutrients in these foods play a crucial role in neurotransmitter function, which is vital for maintaining a calm and balanced state.

2 **Time to Get Moving:** Physical activity, be it brisk walking, dancing, or yoga, releases endorphins, the body's natural mood elevators.

Regular engagement in these activities can significantly enhance mood, reduce anxiety, and improve overall mental health. Finding activities you enjoy will help ensure you make it a habit.

3 **Mindful Practices:** Embracing mindfulness through meditation, mindful eating, and a focus on the now anchors us to the present moment and helps alleviate worries about the past or the future. By focusing on what we are doing right now, we also learn to observe our thoughts and feelings without judgment, leading to a deeper understanding of ourselves and a reduction in stress. Additional practices can include journaling, which allows for reflection and mindfulness through writing, further enhancing emotional awareness and resilience.

4 **Back to Nature:** Time spent outdoors, among trees or by the water, can be incredibly grounding, offering a natural antidote to anxiety. The practice of *forest bathing*, for example, which means spending time in a natural environment, helps you to relax. Waves and waterfalls release negative ions, which can ease stress. Engaging in activities like hiking, gardening, or simply taking a walk in the park can significantly boost your mood, improve your physical health, and strengthen your connection to the natural world.

5 **Connecting and Sharing:** Opening up to loved ones or joining support groups creates a shared space of understanding and compassion. This act of vulnerability can foster deeper connections, reduce feelings of isolation, and provide emotional support during challenging times. Engaging in community service or volunteer work can also offer a sense of purpose and belonging, further enhancing feelings of connectedness and serenity.

6 Restorative Sleep: Sleep isn't just about physical rest. It's a sanctuary for emotional healing. Prioritizing sleep can be one of the best gifts you give yourself. Establishing a soothing bedtime routine, such as reading or taking a warm bath, can prepare your mind and body for rest, enhancing the quality of your sleep. Keeping electronic devices away from the bedroom can also improve sleep hygiene, leading to more restorative sleep and better emotional health.

7 Limit Stimulants: Excess caffeine or sugar can jolt our nervous system, making emotions harder to manage. Moderation is key. Understanding your body's response to these substances and limiting intake can prevent mood swings and promote a more balanced emotional state. Opting for healthier alternatives, such as herbal teas or natural sweeteners like stevia, can also help to improve emotional and physical health.

8 Self-Compassion: Embracing yourself with understanding and love during this turbulent time is paramount. It's like having an internal soothing voice, guiding you with gentleness. Practicing self-compassion involves treating yourself with the same kindness and care you would offer a friend, recognizing that imperfection is part of the human experience. This approach can lead to increased resilience, a more positive self-image, and a greater capacity to navigate life's challenges with grace.

Sleep Deprivation: Creating a Recipe for Restful Sleep

As hormone levels fluctuate, so too does the ability to fall asleep and stay asleep, leading to restless nights and days marked by exhaustion.

HOW TO . . .

Stop Feeling Overwhelmed with Box Breathing

Embrace the simplicity of box breathing for a moment of calm. Inhale for four counts, hold for four counts, and then exhale for four counts, releasing tension. Hold once more for four counts. With each cycle, allow the rhythm of your breath to anchor you, soothe stress, and turn anxiety into stillness.

Understanding the unique interplay between menopause and sleep is the first step toward reducing its effects. Adjusting your bedtime routine, incorporating relaxation techniques, understanding the role of diet and exercise, and adding self-care will help you curate a sleep environment that invites relaxation and restoration.

1 Consistency Is Key: Establish a regular sleep-wake cycle. Waking up and going to sleep at the same time each day, even on the weekends, helps reset your internal clock, keeping it in rhythm much like tuning a well-played instrument. This regularity not only enhances the quality of your sleep but also improves your ability to fall asleep faster.

2 Food, Drink, and Sleep: Caffeine and large meals are notorious for disrupting sleep. It's essential to strike a balance, ensuring your last meal isn't too close to bedtime and is light on the stomach. Eating a heavy meal close to bedtime can affect the release of hormones that regulate sleep, such as melatonin. The presence of certain foods and the process of digestion can interfere with the natural release patterns of these hormones, disrupting your body's internal clock or circadian rhythm (the twenty-four-hour cycle of your internal clock).

3 Sleep Environment: Our bedrooms should be tranquil retreats, free from electronic distractions and excessive brightness. Create a serene sanctuary that helps lull you into a peaceful sleep by using soft, calming colors and comfortable bedding. The temperature of your room can also affect sleep quality, with cooler temperatures generally being more conducive to sleep. Consider the use of blackout curtains or an eye mask to block out any disruptive light, creating an optimal environment for rest.

4 Daily Sunlight Exposure: Embrace the sunlight, the natural regulator of your sleep-wake cycle. Think of it as nature's own energy booster, aligning your circadian rhythm. Regular exposure to natural daylight, especially in the morning, can help maintain a healthy sleep-wake cycle, making it easier to fall asleep and wake up feeling refreshed. Try to spend at least thirty minutes outside each day, whether it's a morning walk or simply enjoying your coffee in the sunshine.

5 Mindful Relaxation: Creating a pre-sleep routine helps to reduce stress and signals your body that it's time to rest. For this reason, choose practices that calm the mind, whether it's deep breathing, meditation, or journaling those racing thoughts—like emptying an overflowing thought jar. When you set aside time each evening to engage in these relaxation techniques, it creates a mental buffer between the day's activities and the quiet of night.

6 A Baby's Sleep Blueprint: Remember the gentle care with which we lull babies to sleep? Adopt a similar nurturing approach for yourself. After all, self-care isn't indulgent—it's vital. This might include a warm bath before bed, a soothing skincare routine, or gentle stretches that signal to your body it's time to rest. Emulating the patience and tenderness we show to infants can help us approach our sleep with the same care, acknowledging its importance in our overall health regimen.

While menopause may challenge your sleep routines, it also presents an opportunity to reimagine your bedtime rituals. With understanding, self-compassion, and deliberate strategies, we can beckon a restful night's sleep and wake up feeling rejuvenated. Sleep isn't merely a necessity, it's the

HOW TO . . .
Get a Good Night's Sleep

Leave your cell phone out of the bedroom. Instead, invest in a classic alarm clock to gently wake you up. Inform your loved ones that your home phone number is to be used only for emergencies after a specific time, or set your phone so you only receive emergency calls after bedtime. These small changes pave the way for uninterrupted tranquility, ensuring your nights are reserved for restful sleep without the temptation of technology.

foundation of your physical condition. Embrace it, prioritize it, and cherish it.

Low Libido: Strategies to Boost Libido and Counteract Vaginal Dryness

1 **Vaginal Moisturizers and Lubricants:** When using over-the-counter vaginal moisturizers, it is beneficial to apply them on a regular basis, not just before sexual activity, to effectively maintain vaginal moisture. This consistent use helps in gradually improving the vaginal tissue's natural moisture levels, offering relief from the discomfort associated with dryness.

When choosing water-based, fragrance-free lubricants for immediate relief, consider selecting products specifically designed for sensitive skin, which further reduces the risk of irritation. Additionally, it's a good practice to apply the lubricant a few minutes before intercourse begins, allowing for the product to adequately coat the area, enhancing comfort and reducing friction right from the start.

2 **Regular Sexual Activity:** It may seem contradictory but engaging in regular sexual activity can help in maintaining vaginal health. Regular sexual activity not only helps stimulate natural lubrication but also improves blood flow to the vaginal area, which can enhance tissue health and elasticity.

To facilitate this, engaging in ample foreplay can increase arousal and natural lubrication, making sexual activity more comfortable and enjoyable. Additionally, staying hydrated and maintaining a balanced diet rich in phytoestrogens and omega-3 fatty acids can support vaginal health from the inside out, further promoting natural lubrication.

3 **Phytoestrogens:** These are natural occurring compounds found in certain foods that mimic estrogen in the body that help in alleviating some menopausal symptoms. Incorporating foods rich in phytoestrogens, such as flaxseeds, sesame seeds, legumes, and soy products helps support hormonal balance during menopause.

To optimize the intake of these beneficial compounds, consider adding them to your daily meals in creative ways, such as blending flaxseeds into smoothies or using soy milk in your morning cereal. This not only enhances your diet's nutritional profile but also ensures a steady supply of natural phytoestrogens to help mitigate menopausal symptoms effectively.

4 **Pelvic Floor Exercises:** Exercises to help strengthen the pelvic floor can help enhance sexual pleasure and maintain pelvic floor health. This area is often neglected in workouts, but just because you can't see the results in the mirror doesn't mean you shouldn't work on it! To effectively strengthen the pelvic floor, you need to contract and relax the pelvic floor muscles. This can be done almost anywhere and at any time.

Pilates and yoga also engage and strengthen the pelvic floor muscles through a series of focused movements and poses and improve overall strength and flexibility. Integrating these exercises into your workout not only enhances pelvic floor health but also contributes to better posture and core stability.

5 **Mindfulness Meditation CBT Therapy:** Mindfulness meditation and cognitive behavioral therapy (CBT) have shown promise in addressing low libido in menopausal women and help to manage stress too. To incorporate mindfulness meditation into your routine, start with short

daily sessions focusing on your breath or a specific object, gradually increasing the duration as you become more comfortable with the practice. This can help reduce stress and increase awareness of your body's sensations, enhancing emotional connectivity during sexual intimacy.

CBT can help you to identify and change negative thought patterns and beliefs about sexuality, aging, and menopause that may be impacting your libido. Engaging in CBT can also provide strategies for improving communication with your partner, further enriching the emotional and intimate aspects of your relationship.

6 **Open Communication:** It can be beneficial to discuss your feelings and concerns about the changes you're experiencing with your partner. The more you stay silent, the more your partner may feel rejected. So, communication is key. Setting aside dedicated time for open and honest discussions with your partner about the changes you're experiencing can create a supportive environment for both of you to express your feelings and concerns. This can involve sharing personal experiences, fears, and desires, which can help in setting realistic expectations and finding mutual ground to reignite the spark in your relationship.

Couple's therapy that focuses on improving intimacy can be beneficial. You may also want to engage in an activity as a couple, such as regular date nights that create closeness or attending a workshop or session on improving sexual communication and connection. All these activities can help strengthen your bond and enable you to navigate menopausal changes together.

Know that you are not alone. A low libido is not your fault or something to be embarrassed about. The more we talk, the more we normalize this

CARA'S FAVORITE WAY TO . . .

Get in the Mood

Sometimes, the more we dwell on the idea of intimacy, the more reasons we find to avoid it, especially if we're not immediately feeling amorous. The key is to sidestep overthinking and embrace the Nike philosophy, "Just Do It." Keep your favorite lubricant within easy reach and let spontaneity lead the way. You might just find that your hesitance gives way to an unexpected and enjoyable encounter.

change and the easier it is to move through and past it. Your relationship will grow stronger, and you'll feel more empowered as you share your experience.

Less Common Menopause Symptoms

Menopause marks a significant transition in a woman's life, commonly associated with well-known symptoms such as hot flashes and night sweats. However, this period can also bring about a host of lesser-known symptoms that can be just as impactful but are often not discussed as frequently. These symptoms can affect a woman's quality of life in various ways, ranging from physical discomforts to changes in sensory perceptions and emotional state.

Understanding these lesser-known symptoms is crucial when you're navigating this phase of life. It helps to validate what you're experiencing and helps you find solutions.

Lesser-Known Menopause Symptoms

SYMPTOM	DESCRIPTION	SOLUTION
Burning Mouth Syndrome	This is a sensation of burning in the tongue, lips, gums, or other areas of the mouth without an apparent medical cause.	Avoid spicy and acidic foods that can exacerbate the burning sensation, common during menopause due to hormonal fluctuations.
Electric Shock Sensation	Some women report feeling a sudden, sharp electric shock sensation, primarily in the head or the layers of tissue under the skin, often as a precursor to a hot flash.	Increase your intake of omega-3 fatty acids, which can help stabilize nerve cell membranes and potentially reduce these sensations during menopause.
Tingling Extremities	Tingling sensations in the hands, feet, arms, and legs can occur due to hormonal changes affecting the nervous system.	Engage in regular, moderate exercise to improve circulation and reduce the occurrence of tingling, often linked to menopausal hormonal changes.
Gum Problems	Hormonal fluctuations can lead to dry mouth, increased sensitivity, and a greater risk of gum disease.	Use a softer toothbrush and consider saliva-promoting products to combat dry mouth, a condition that can worsen with menopause.
Change in Body Odor	Alterations in hormone levels can lead to changes in body odor during menopause.	Apply natural mineral salts or crystal deodorant, which can be more effective in managing the change in body odor associated with menopause.
Dizziness and Balance Issues	Some women may experience dizziness or a feeling of being off-balance, not linked to vertigo or inner ear disorders.	Practice yoga, tai chi, or similar balance-enhancing exercises, as hormonal shifts during menopause can affect your equilibrium.
Vision Changes	Hormonal adjustments during menopause can lead to changes in vision, including dry eyes, fluctuating visual acuity, and increased sensitivity to light. These changes can impact overall eye comfort and may necessitate adjustments in eyewear prescriptions or the use of lubricating eye drops.	Increase room humidity and take frequent screen breaks to combat dry eyes, a common issue as estrogen levels drop during menopause.
Breast Pain	Hormonal changes can cause breast soreness or tenderness, which is not limited to the premenopausal phase.	Apply evening primrose oil topically or consume it in capsule form, as it contains gamma-linolenic acid (GLA), which may help balance hormones and alleviate breast tenderness in menopausal women.
Digestive Problems	Fluctuating hormones can affect the digestive tract, leading to symptoms like bloating, stomach pain, and changes in bowel habits.	Incorporate probiotic-rich foods like yogurt into your diet to support gut health, as digestive issues can become more pronounced with the hormonal changes of menopause.
Onset of Allergies	New allergies or an increase in allergic reactions can occur, possibly due to the immune system's response to hormonal changes.	Consider using a high-efficiency particulate air (HEPA) filter in your home to remove allergens from the air, as menopause can sometimes heighten sensitivity to environmental allergens.

You Can Do This!

Menopause, with its many challenges, also offers an opportunity for renewal and improved self-confidence and emotional well-being. With knowledge, self-care, and support, you can navigate the emotional landscape of menopause one step at a time with resilience and grace. Remember, this is a shared journey, and we're in it together!

Action Steps

1 **Write out a seven-day food diary.** It will help you become more aware of how your diet is affecting each menopause symptom.

2 **After seven days,** evaluate your diary and see where you can make simple changes.

3 **Clear your kitchen cupboards** of all processed foods. Think about adding more natural whole foods, and if your pocketbook allows, organic foods.

4 **Buy a large water bottle,** fill it, and always keep it with you. Drink when your mouth feels dry.

5 **Look ahead to the recipes** in part 3 and plan your meals for one week. You'll be eating delicious, healthy foods that are designed to reduce menopausal symptoms and help you feel better.

4

Why Blood Sugar Balance Matters and How to Get Off of the Blood Sugar Roller Coaster

You might be surprised to know that the root of many menopausal symptoms can be traced back to fluctuations in blood glucose levels, which can exacerbate hormonal changes. This can make you feel even worse. Erratic glucose (sugar) levels can intensify hot flashes, mood swings, weight gain, and sleep disturbances.

The foods you consume directly impact your blood sugar levels, and by extension, your hormonal balance. This means you need to begin to choose foods and eat in a way that stabilizes blood sugar levels. Proper nutrition is not just a supplementary aid, it's essential for managing menopause effectively. Consider it the foundation upon which all other efforts are built.

Blood Sugar and Its Domino Effect on Hormones

Imagine this: You skip a meal or perhaps indulge in a sugary treat, causing a rapid spike and subsequent crash in your blood sugar levels. Your body, ever the protective guardian, perceives this dip as a threat. Its immediate response is to release cortisol and adrenaline, our "fight or flight" hormones. These hormones surge to quickly raise blood sugar levels, ensuring your brain and body have the essential energy they need to function.

Simultaneously, these dips often trigger intense cravings for sugary foods. It's not a lack of willpower. It's a physiological response. The body is simply trying to get a quick energy source to counteract the drop in blood sugar. When you give in to these cravings, you inadvertently cause another spike in blood sugar, only for it to crash again later. This becomes a relentless roller coaster ride of peaks and lows.

THE ADRENAL GLANDS: CAUGHT IN THE CROSSFIRE

Our adrenal glands, which are instrumental in producing cortisol in response to stress, serve as a backup system for estrogen production during menopause. If you're continuously engaged in managing these blood sugar crises, the ability to produce estrogen effectively diminishes.

It's a chain reaction. Erratic blood sugar leads to adrenal fatigue, which in turn compromises estrogen production. And as we've established, a dip in estrogen can heighten menopausal symptoms. The cycle, once set in motion, can feel relentless and exhausting.

BREAKING THE CYCLE

Balancing your blood sugar isn't just a strategy. It's a lifeline. By ensuring consistent energy levels and

Client Success Story

I counted calories for years religiously (a bit too obsessively). It always worked for me until I turned fifty. After that, I started to gain weight no matter how few calories I had. Learning to focus on my nutrition and balancing my blood sugar levels and to not worry so much about calories hasn't been easy, but I promised myself that I would trust the process. Unbelievably, the weight came off, and I no longer stress about my calories. I am thrilled with my results. Thank you, Cara!

—CHRISTINA

reducing the strain on your adrenal glands, you're giving your body the grace to navigate menopause with greater ease.

THE BODY'S BACKUP SYSTEM: THE ADRENAL GLANDS

Let's take a closer look at why blood sugar balance is so pivotal when it comes to easing menopausal symptoms, estrogen's role in regulating blood glucose levels, and your adrenal glands. The human body is a master of intricate systems, all interwoven to ensure equilibrium. This balance is particularly important when it comes to your hormones.

THE ROLE OF ADRENAL GLANDS IN ESTROGEN PRODUCTION

The adrenal glands are nothing short of amazing. These tiny glands, positioned neatly above your kidneys, are your hormonal safety net. As we've seen, as ovarian estrogen production dwindles, the adrenal glands step up, producing a weaker form of estrogen to help maintain a semblance of your hormonal balance. However, this backup system comes with its own set of challenges, specifically stress and how we react to it.

THE MIDLIFE STRESS CONUNDRUM

Midlife is often painted as a time of tranquility and reflection, but for many people, it's anything but. It's more like juggling on a tightrope. Children no matter their age still turn to you, elderly parents need care, demanding jobs consume your days, households demand attention, and in the middle of all of this, you're trying your best to maintain all your relationships. Such multifaceted stress is not just an emotional or mental burden, it physically impacts your body, especially your adrenal glands.

THE OVERBURDENED ADRENAL GLANDS

Your adrenal glands, in their effort to keep up with the demands of your hectic life, frequently pump out stress hormones. This constant production can take its toll. Remember, these are the same glands you're relying on to produce estrogen as a backup during menopause. If they're overwhelmed by stress, their efficiency in hormone regulation, including estrogen production, wanes.

THE STRESS CONNECTION: ADRENALS, ESTROGEN, AND BLOOD SUGAR BALANCE

When you experience stress, the adrenal glands release cortisol, a hormone that's designed to help you fight or flee. When cortisol levels rise, it stimulates the liver to produce glucose from non-carbohydrate sources through a process called gluconeogenesis, which makes the body more resistant to insulin. This ensures that more glucose is available in the bloodstream to provide energy quickly. However, if cortisol levels remain high over a prolonged period, this can also lead to consistently elevated blood sugar levels.

Stress, in all its forms, directly impacts your adrenal glands' capacity to function optimally. If these glands are constantly preoccupied with managing high cortisol levels due to stressors, their ability to produce estrogen diminishes.

Balancing blood sugar isn't just about managing energy levels or weight. It's intricately tied to how our body navigates the hormonal changes of menopause. By understanding and respecting the interplay of hormones, it's easier to find solutions and better equip yourself to sail smoothly through this life transition.

Menopause 101

There are three types of estrogen:

1 **Estrone (E1):** After menopause and during perimenopause, your body's primary estrogen is estrone, predominantly produced by the adipose (fat) tissues and your adrenal glands.

2 **Estradiol (E2):** During your reproductive years, estradiol is the main form of estrogen, mainly synthesized in the ovaries. It's known for being the most potent estrogen type.

3 **Estriol (E3):** In pregnancy, estriol becomes the primary estrogen, produced largely by the placenta. It plays an essential role in supporting the pregnancy.

Stress Caused by Perimenopause and Menopause

That's not all. Perimenopause and menopause are transitional stages in a woman's life, with hormonal fluctuations that cause even more stress, impacting almost every system in the body. This stress involves every aspect of the hypothalamic-pituitary-adrenal (HPA) axis, a complex network of interactions between three glands: the hypothalamus, the pituitary, and the adrenal glands, which also affects blood sugar balance.

Our bodies are marvels of interconnected systems. The HPA axis, pivotal in managing stress and hormonal balance, plays a significant role during the menopausal transition. Recognizing its importance and understanding its function allows us to make informed decisions, particularly regarding stress management and hormonal balance, during these transformative years.

Did You Know?

The three glands in the HPA axis are as follows:

1 **Hypothalamus:** Located in the brain, the hypothalamus is responsible for maintaining the body's internal balance. It oversees various bodily functions such as temperature, hunger, and thirst. When the hypothalamus detects an imbalance—for example, high levels of stress—it sends a signal to the pituitary gland.

2 **Pituitary Gland:** Often referred to as the "master gland," the pituitary receives instructions from the hypothalamus and then releases hormones that act on other glands and tissues. In response to stress, it secretes the adrenocorticotropic hormone (ACTH).

3 **Adrenal Glands:** Situated atop our kidneys, the adrenal glands are the final responders in this chain. They receive ACTH from the pituitary and release the stress hormone cortisol, along with other hormones. Among these is a weak form of estrogen, especially crucial during the menopausal transition when ovarian estrogen production declines.

THE HPA AXIS AND MENOPAUSE

During perimenopause and menopause, the HPA axis plays a crucial role in maintaining hormonal balance. Normally, the HPA axis ensures the body's equilibrium, but as estrogen production declines with menopause, the adrenal glands partially take over this hormone's production.

This transition could be smooth, but it becomes complicated with prolonged stress. Stress demands constant cortisol production from the adrenal glands, which not only raises blood sugar levels as a direct stress response but also diverts the glands' resources away from producing estrogen.

This scenario creates a double-edged sword for menopausal women. On one hand, elevated cortisol levels due to stress lead to higher blood sugar levels, contributing to the risk of insulin resistance and metabolic issues. On the other hand, the adrenal glands, burdened by cortisol production, can't compensate for the body's declining estrogen, exacerbating menopausal symptoms like hot flashes, mood swings, and sleep disturbances. Moreover, balanced estrogen levels are crucial for insulin sensitivity and glucose metabolism, indicating that estrogen's diminished production can indirectly contribute to blood sugar imbalances.

Therefore, managing stress and supporting adrenal health becomes paramount in balancing blood sugar during menopause. Strategies to mitigate stress, such as mindfulness meditation, moderate exercise, and adequate rest, can help stabilize cortisol levels, thereby aiding in maintaining both hormonal balance and blood sugar levels. This holistic approach ensures that the adrenal glands are not overtaxed, supporting their role in estrogen production and contributing to a smoother menopausal transition while also addressing blood sugar regulation challenges.

CHRONIC STRESS AND WEIGHT GAIN: THE HORMONAL LINK

As chronic stress results in the overproduction of cortisol, estrogen produced by the ovaries declines. This drop signals to the body that it needs more, and in its infinite wisdom and drive to maintain equilibrium, finds alternative sources. The first stop is the adrenal glands, but as they become over-worked, it looks for another source.

THE UNWANTED GUEST: MENOPAUSAL BELLY FAT

Menopause, while a natural and inevitable phase in a woman's life, often brings with it challenges that many weren't prepared for. One of the most prevalent and disconcerting is the sudden accumulation of belly fat.

Fat cells, especially those around the abdomen, can produce estrogen. So, when your body seeks to increase its declining estrogen levels, it often responds by increasing the number of these estrogen-producing fat cells, leading to the dreaded belly fat. The body's intention is noble—it's trying to help by naturally boosting estrogen—but this "solution" can feel anything but helpful.

THE VICIOUS CYCLE OF STRESS AND BELLY FAT

Gaining belly fat can be distressing, affecting your self-esteem and confidence. Many women describe feeling "out of sync" with their bodies during this time and are frustrated by the sudden change. This emotional turmoil can, in turn, increase stress levels, leading to even more cortisol production and further reinforcing the cycle of stress and weight gain.

Moreover, the general advice to "eat less and exercise more" isn't a magic bullet here. Visceral fat, the type of fat that accumulates around the abdomen, doesn't respond only to a caloric deficit. Its roots are hormonal, which means addressing it requires a holistic approach that factors in the complex hormonal interplays at work.

Small Steps, Big Results

Dedicating just ten minutes a day to meditation can lead to amazing shifts in your stress levels, which can, in turn, positively influence weight management during menopause. As you embark on the practice of meditation, allow yourself to fully trust in its life-altering power. With consistent practice, you're likely to discover profound and gratifying changes in both your physical and mental well-being. Embrace meditation as a gentle yet powerful tool in your journey through menopause. You'll find guided meditations in part 2.

Understanding Insulin and Insulin Resistance: Key Players in Blood Sugar Regulation

So far, you've learned how shifting and dipping hormone levels cause menopause symptoms and how important blood sugar regulation is in reducing them. Insulin is the most important hormone when it comes to blood sugar levels. So, it's important to understand insulin's role and something called *insulin resistance*, which means the body can't use this hormone effectively to balance blood sugar levels. Together, insulin and insulin resistance play pivotal roles in the balance of blood sugar levels and how you feel during menopause.

THE INSULIN MECHANISM: BALANCER OF BLOOD SUGAR

Your body operates within an intricate framework designed to maintain balance, especially when it comes to blood sugar levels. Imagine blood sugar as a Goldilocks zone: too high or too low and your body perceives a state of emergency. Consuming foods rich in sugars or refined carbohydrates, like white bread, cakes, pastries, white pasta, or many processed breakfast cereals, catapults your blood sugar to levels higher than your body deems ideal. Enter insulin.

Insulin, often termed the "key" to our cells, springs into action when it's released from the pancreas when it detects this surge. It's like a traffic cop, directing the excess glucose from your bloodstream to various destinations, such as your liver, muscles, and other cells, so it's absorbed and used for energy.

However, as with any system, there's a limit to how much it can do. When your cells are inundated with too much sugar, much like an overstuffed suitcase, and can't take in anymore, the excess gets converted and stored as fat.

Fat cells, especially those located in the abdominal area, play a more complex role in the body's endocrine system than previously understood. Beyond their function as storage units for excess energy, these adipose tissues (belly fat) are metabolically active and capable of producing and releasing estrogen into the bloodstream.

This adaptation can have unintended consequences. The estrogen produced by fat cells can contribute to a cycle that exacerbates menopausal symptoms and leads to further health complications. For example, higher levels of estrogen derived from adipose tissue can lead to increased fat accumulation, particularly in the abdominal area, creating a feedback loop that can aggravate symptoms such as weight gain, hot flashes, and mood swings.

THE AFTERMATH: THE SUGAR CRASH AND ITS REPERCUSSIONS

Once insulin does its job, there's a significant drop in your blood sugar levels, often plunging it below the ideal range. This crash manifests in feelings of fatigue, anxiety, irritability, and dizziness. It feels like an energy bankruptcy, leaving you desperate for a quick fix and triggers the release of cortisol and adrenaline. As you've seen, cortisol can create potent cravings, compelling you to reach for those same high-sugar, processed foods. So, the cycle repeats.

INSULIN RESISTANCE: A LOCKED DOOR

Over time, with continuous exposure to high sugar levels, your cells grow weary. Imagine constantly knocking on a door and demanding someone take more and more deliveries when they're already overwhelmed. Eventually, they'll probably stop answering. Similarly, to protect themselves, your cells become less responsive to insulin's knocks. This is called *insulin resistance*. As cells reject more and more sugar, it's then stored as fat, which can accumulate around our midsection.

Menopause 101

During menopause, the body goes through significant hormonal changes that can affect insulin sensitivity. Substances like alcohol, caffeine, and nicotine are known to influence insulin response, which can exacerbate menopausal symptoms such as weight fluctuation and hot flashes. Moderating your intake of these substances can help stabilize insulin levels, potentially easing these symptoms. Mindful consumption is particularly beneficial during menopause, as it supports your body's changing needs and contributes to overall hormonal balance.

What's the crux of the matter? Relying heavily on high-sugar and processed foods doesn't just spike your blood sugar, it sets off a ripple effect of events, exacerbating weight gain, especially around the belly, and complicating the already-delicate hormonal balance during menopause. Focusing on quality nutrition and understanding the mechanics of your body's response to food can pave the way for better health decisions during this critical phase of life.

As you can see, blood sugar regulation is an intricate process that involves a series of players, each with their role and responsibility. Understanding insulin and insulin resistance helps you grasp the deeper implications of your dietary choices, especially during menopause. This knowledge equips you to make empowered decisions as you seek to balance your blood sugar levels and navigate the menopausal transition with grace.

BALANCING BLOOD SUGAR: A STRESS-RELIEF LEVER

To sum up, while it might seem counterintuitive to link blood sugar with stress, the connection is clear and scientifically based. Stress affects blood sugar levels and vice versa. Erratic blood sugar levels, particularly those resulting from consuming

---

HOW TO . . .

Understand Insulin Resistance with Cara's Spring Break Analogy

Picture your youthful twenties, filled with the adventurous spirit of Spring Break: Feasting, toasting, and very little sleep, yet you recover swiftly, your vitality seemingly boundless. Your body adeptly manages these indulgences, both in stamina and spirit.

Leap to your thirties, and the Spring Break saga takes a twist. Attempting to echo the carefree escapades of your younger years, you find the rebound isn't as quick. A full day of revelry leaves you lagging, the once-easy bounce back now a trudge.

Now, envision your forties, where the plot thickens. The same old routine of minimal rest, too much alcohol, and fast-food feasts now exacts a stiffer price. Enter the diligent pancreas, working hard to pump out insulin to purge the sugar from your system. But this time, your muscles and organs are less cooperative, declining insulin's attempts to do its job. As a result, your fat cells become an all-too-eager refuge, expanding as they stockpile the surplus.

This analogy underscores the progressive nature of insulin resistance, which is similar to how our recovery from youthful indulgences diminishes with age. Just as the body struggles more with each decade to bounce back from the excesses of Spring Break, it similarly faces increasing difficulty in managing blood sugar levels due to insulin resistance. Recognizing this shift is crucial for implementing lifestyle changes, such as improved diet and increased exercise, to help maintain metabolic health and prevent further complications.

sugar-laden foods, induce stress in the body, leading to elevated cortisol levels. When blood sugar spikes after indulging in sugary treats, it inevitably crashes soon after, which the body interprets as a stress event, prompting a cortisol release in response.

Incorporating a diet rich in whole foods, including complex carbohydrates like whole grains, legumes, and vegetables, can stabilize blood sugar levels. These foods are digested more slowly, providing a gradual release of sugar into the bloodstream, which helps maintain steady energy levels and mood. Additionally, including quality proteins and healthy fats in your meals can further aid in blood sugar regulation by slowing the absorption of glucose and minimizing spikes and crashes.

While life might not offer the luxury of eliminating stress, through thoughtful nutrition and effective blood sugar management, you can significantly mitigate its impact on your adrenal glands. This strategic approach to eating not only supports your body's ability to maintain hormonal balance but also enhances your overall resilience to daily stressors. It allows your adrenal glands to function more optimally, producing estrogen, and manage other stressors with greater efficiency. By prioritizing a balanced diet, you empower your body to navigate the challenges of stress with more stability and vigor.

Nutrition: Your First Line of Defense

So, how do you keep your blood sugar levels stable? The answer lies in your diet and eating foods with a low glycemic index (a score given to food depending on how much it raises blood sugar levels), which are a mix of lean protein, healthy fats, and complex carbohydrates. In addition, being mindful of *what* you eat and *when* (meal timings) can all contribute to stabilized blood sugar. This dietary approach doesn't just benefit your energy levels. It's a direct

HOW TO . . .

Balance Blood Sugar by Getting Rid of Processed Foods

To reduce menopause symptoms, it's best to focus on whole, unprocessed foods that don't come prepackaged or have long shelf lives in supermarkets. Those items are full of preservatives, additives, and emulsifiers to extend their expiration dates, which can be detrimental to your health. By choosing fresh, nutrient-rich foods, you're not only reducing your intake of unnecessary chemicals but also fortifying your body's natural ability to manage menopausal changes. This approach to nutrition is a foundational strategy for enhancing your overall health during the menopausal transition.

and actionable strategy to lessen the burden on your adrenal glands.

MASTERING BLOOD SUGAR LEVELS THROUGH DIET

Stepping off the blood sugar roller coaster might seem like a daunting task, especially when cravings hold a compelling grip. Yet, the knowledge that these dietary fluctuations exacerbate menopausal symptoms should be your compass guiding you towards better choices. You'll learn more about comprehensive strategies regarding food and how it can ease your symptoms in the next chapter, but let's start with foundational elements: complex carbohydrates and proteins.

COMPLEX CARBOHYDRATES: A SUSTAINED ENERGY SOURCE

Complex carbohydrates are like the slow-burning logs in a fireplace, as opposed to the quick-burning paper of simple sugars. Complex carbs provide prolonged, steady energy release, ensuring that your blood sugar doesn't spike sharply after meals.

Examples of Complex Carbohydrates

- **Whole Grains:** Think quinoa, brown rice, barley, and oats. These are unrefined grains, meaning they retain the entirety of their nutrient-rich bran, germ (the nutrient-rich embryo of the grain), and endosperm (the largest part of the grain). Whole grains help in managing blood sugar by providing a steady source of energy and preventing rapid spikes in blood sugar levels, thanks to their high fiber content and complex carbohydrates.

- **Legumes:** Beans, lentils, and chickpeas not only offer carbohydrates but also pack a protein punch, which is great for satiety, keeping you full for longer. This will help stop cravings for simple carbohydrates, responsible for spiking and crashing your blood sugar levels. All of these also contain phytoestrogens and essential nutrients that help balance hormones.

- **Vegetables:** Choose nonstarchy ones like broccoli, brussels sprouts, and leafy greens. Their fiber content slows down the absorption of sugars into the bloodstream, helping to maintain steady blood sugar levels.

- **Fruits:** Opt for whole fruits rather than fruit juices. Berries, apples (with the skin), and pears are particularly high in fiber, beneficial for reducing menopause symptoms and balancing blood sugar because the fiber helps slow down glucose absorption, preventing spikes in blood sugar, while also supporting hormonal balance and digestive health, alleviating menopause-related discomforts.

Reasons to Embrace Them

- **Steady Energy Release:** The fiber content of these foods means they're digested slower, providing a consistent energy source, which avoids blood sugar peaks and valleys.

- **Nutrient-Dense:** Complex carbs often contain essential vitamins and minerals beneficial for overall health.

- **Satiety:** The fiber in complex carbs adds bulk to your meals, making you feel fuller for longer.

PROTEIN: THE BUILDING BLOCKS OF LIFE

Proteins play an indispensable role in the maintenance and functioning of our bodies, serving as the foundational building blocks of life. They are essential for nearly every cellular process, from repairing damaged tissues and muscles to synthesizing the enzymes that facilitate countless biochemical reactions. This vital nutrient not only supports physical health and recovery but also contributes to the efficient operation of our metabolic and immune systems, underscoring the importance of incorporating adequate protein into our diets for physical fitness and vitality.

Examples of Protein Sources

- **Animal-Based:** Sources like chicken, turkey, fish, lean beef, and eggs are pivotal in a balanced diet because they provide complete proteins.

This means they contain all essential amino acids, which are the building blocks your body cannot synthesize on its own and must obtain from food. Essential amino acids play critical roles in muscle repair, hormone production, and overall bodily functions, making animal-based proteins crucial for maintaining muscle mass, supporting recovery, and ensuring that the body operates smoothly.

- **Plant-Based:** Lentils, black beans, chickpeas, tofu, tempeh, and edamame are excellent plant-based sources of protein. While many plant proteins are not complete, meaning they don't contain all essential amino acids, consuming a variety of plant-based proteins can ensure you receive all necessary amino acids over time.

  An added benefit of plant-based proteins is their content of complex carbohydrates. These carbohydrates are important because they provide a sustained energy source, help regulate blood sugar levels, and are rich in fiber, which supports digestive health and can aid in weight management. The presence of fiber and other nutrients in plant-based proteins also contributes to a feeling of fullness, which can help with appetite control.

- **Dairy and Alternatives:** Greek yogurt, cottage cheese, and various cheeses offer high-quality protein and are excellent sources of calcium and other vital nutrients. For individuals who are lactose intolerant or choose to avoid dairy for other reasons, alternatives like almond milk, soy milk, or pea protein powder are beneficial. These alternatives not only provide protein but also are often fortified with other nutrients such as calcium, vitamin D, and vitamin B12, which might be lacking in a dairy-free diet. This makes them an essential part of a balanced diet, ensuring that those who avoid dairy still receive necessary nutrients for bone health, muscle function, and overall well-being.

In summary, proteins, whether from animal, plant, or dairy sources, are essential for numerous bodily functions, including growth, repair, and the maintenance of good health. The diversity of protein sources available allows individuals to choose options that fit their dietary preferences and nutritional needs, ensuring they can obtain all essential amino acids and benefit from the additional nutrients these foods offer.

Reasons to Incorporate Protein

- **Stabilizes Blood Sugar:** Protein has a negligible effect on blood sugar levels and can help regulate the rate at which carbohydrates are digested and absorbed, leading to a more controlled and gradual rise in blood sugar.

- **Satiety:** Protein's ability to promote satiety can significantly reduce the urge to snack between meals, aiding in weight management. This effect is due to protein's slow digestion and its impact on hunger hormones, which together prolong the feeling of fullness. Consequently, incorporating protein-rich foods into your diet can help curb unnecessary snacking, a common contributor to weight gain, by keeping you satisfied for longer periods and supporting healthier eating habits.

- **Supports Muscle Mass:** As we age, it becomes increasingly important to maintain muscle mass not only for strength but also for metabolic health, as muscles significantly influence metabolism. Adequate protein intake is vital for muscle preservation because it supplies the essential amino acids needed for muscle repair and growth. Insufficient protein can lead to muscle loss and a slower metabolic rate, complicating weight management and raising the risk of metabolic disorders. Ensuring enough protein in the diet is crucial to support a healthy metabolism and maintain muscle mass in older adults.

THE MAGIC OF COMBINING THE RIGHT FOODS

When you combine lean protein, fiber, and complex carbohydrates in your meals, you not only provide your body with balanced nutrition but also help regulate your blood sugar levels, which eases menopausal symptoms. The slow-release energy from the carbs paired with the stabilizing effect of protein and fiber ensures that your blood sugar remains within a steady range post-meals.

STEPPING OFF THE BLOOD SUGAR ROLLER COASTER: ADD BEFORE YOU SUBTRACT

It's human nature to be drawn toward the very thing you're told to resist! When you label certain foods as "forbidden," we want them more. So, instead of focusing just on what you can't eat, take a moment to shift your perspective and think about nourishment rather than deprivation. Instead of stripping away, let's layer in the goodness. This subtle shift can make the journey of balancing blood sugar more approachable and sustainable.

So, before diving headfirst into what should be reduced or eliminated, let's focus on what can be added. Here are some key strategies:

1 **Boost Your Fiber Intake:** Incorporate more fiber-rich foods like chia seeds, flaxseeds, broccoli, berries, and whole grains into your diet. These not only help you feel fuller for longer but also ensure a steady release of energy, and the high fiber content aids in digestion and can reduce the risk of chronic diseases.

2 **Prioritize Healthy Fats:** Add avocados, nuts such as almonds, walnuts, pecans, and cashews, seeds like chia, flax, pumpkin, and sesame, as well as olive oil to your meals. These sources of healthy fats not only keep you satiated but also help stabilize blood sugar levels, contributing to heart health and reducing inflammation.

3 **Hydrate with Purpose:** Choose water infused with cucumber, lemon, or mint over sugary drinks. This switch to refreshing alternatives can fulfill your desire for flavored beverages without leading to a sugar spike, promoting better hydration and overall health.

4 **Spice It Up:** Utilize cinnamon, which has been shown to help regulate blood sugar levels. Adding it to your morning oatmeal or coffee can provide a flavorful twist and health benefits, including antioxidant properties and blood sugar regulation.

5 **Lean on Protein:** Protein is crucial for satiety and managing blood sugar. Ensure you include a serving of protein at every meal, whether it's from lean meats, legumes, or dairy products, to support muscle maintenance and energy levels throughout the day.

SHIFT YOUR MINDSET

So, instead of focusing on the "I can't have," shift your mindset to "Look at what I get to have!" Focus on adding vibrant colors to your plate, diverse textures, and most importantly, dense nutrients that fuel the body. With this approach, you'll soon find that the foods you once craved, those high in sugar or overly processed, might just lose their appeal naturally as you feel more satisfied and energized with your nutrient-dense choices.

The journey to stepping off the blood sugar roller coaster isn't about stringent rules or harsh restrictions. It's about embracing a perspective of abundance, understanding the beneficial impact of every positive food choice we make, and layering in the goodness, bite by bite.

MENOPAUSE AND BLOOD SUGAR BALANCE: NAVIGATING STORMY SEAS

Navigating the landscape of menopause often feels like sailing stormy seas, with hormones ebbing and flowing unpredictably, which can affect blood sugar regulation and subsequently the symptoms you experience.

As we've seen, the blood sugar roller coaster, a cycle of spiking and crashing, can amplify menopausal discomforts. Recognizing the pivotal role of diet, especially the significance of complex carbohydrates and protein, highlights a path to more stable blood sugar levels.

These dietary choices, while straightforward, can deliver remarkable benefits. They offer continuous energy, stabilize your internal systems, and importantly, provide an environment where the adrenal glands can function their best, producing essential estrogen during perimenopause and menopause.

Balancing your blood sugar is key to feeling better during menopause, but it's not just about what you eat. It's about embracing a holistic approach that combines good food with a great mindset. By doing this, you're setting yourself up for a smoother ride through menopause.

As we wrap up this chapter, let's get ready to dive into the next one, where we'll take a closer look at nutrition. We're going to bust the myth that food is the enemy. Instead, we'll see it as the powerful ally it truly is, giving you the energy and support you need to ease those menopause symptoms. It's all about changing how we think about food. So, let's gear up for some positive changes and discover how to make food work for you during menopause.

Action Steps

1 **Take your time.** You're processing lots of new information, which can feel overwhelming.

2 **Understanding the effects** that erratic blood sugar can have on your menopausal symptoms will help you make positive changes that will help you feel better.

3 **Choose three small changes** that you can make this week in your diet.

4 **Remember to drink** whenever your mouth feels dry to stay hydrated.

5 **Add five different fruits** and vegetables to your plate each day.

5

Food Is Not the Enemy

As the twilight years of fertility set in and the dawn of menopause emerges, many of us find ourselves re-evaluating our relationship with food. Often, women view food as the enemy, especially when we gain weight during menopause, but it's not. In fact, when we choose the right foods, we find an ally, a source of nourishment, energy, and balance. In this chapter, you'll rediscover the importance of focusing on food quality, understand its pivotal role in alleviating menopausal symptoms, and shed any associated guilt that you may feel when eating.

Beyond the confines of calories and numbers, food stands as a beacon of nourishment, warmth, and even celebration.

Food is life. It's energy. It's healing. And, most importantly, it's something to be enjoyed, not feared. As you approach and journey through menopause, remember that the quality of what you put into your body will invariably influence how you feel. Let's celebrate food for the incredible friend it can be during this transformative time and recognize its power to comfort, heal, and nourish.

Let's dive in!

Break Free from Calorie Counting During Menopause

When it comes to nutrition during menopause, the age-old mantra of calorie counting just doesn't add up. That's because you need to focus on the nutritional value of what you consume to manage menopausal symptoms.

Much like the intricate workings of insulin within our bodies, the weight management equation extends beyond the basic "calories in versus calories out" model. During menopause, the body undergoes a complex metamorphosis, with its nutritional demands becoming more nuanced and multifaceted.

When you fixate solely on caloric intake, it's like trying to understand a masterpiece painting by looking only at one brushstroke. The broader picture, involving nutrient absorption, hormonal changes, metabolic rate, and more, tends to be missed. Menopause accentuates this, as the body's responses to food evolve, with some processes becoming more pronounced.

THE EMOTIONAL IMPACT OF COUNTING CALORIES

The continual monitoring of calorie consumption doesn't just affect us physically, but emotionally too. Obsessive calorie counting can ruin the innate pleasure and cultural significance of food, turning every meal into a mathematical equation rather than a nourishing experience to be savored.

Further complicating matters, this constant self-surveillance can induce stress. As we've touched upon earlier, stress, especially chronic stress, has its own set of repercussions during menopause. It can also stimulate weight gain, which is completely counterproductive. Instead of feeling conflicted, the food you eat needs to be a source of nourishment, comfort, and celebration, especially during these formative years.

BEYOND CALORIE COUNTING: NURTURING A WHOLESOME RELATIONSHIP WITH FOOD

Food is more than just counting calories. It's a way to nourish our bodies so that we can be our best selves, especially during menopause. When you implement this strategy, you start to eat with more intention and mindfulness, transforming mealtimes into opportunities for connection, reflection, and gratitude.

CHAMPION THE POWER OF NUTRIENT-RICH FOODS

So, instead of focusing on calorie counting, zero in on nutrient-rich foods in every bite you eat. For instance, foods like leafy greens, vibrant berries, crunchy nuts, and seeds are treasure troves of nutrition. They're not just food. They're rich sources of antioxidants, essential fatty acids, vitamins, and minerals. Consuming these superfoods can arm the body with the tools it needs to navigate and alleviate the multifaceted symptoms of menopause.

EMBARK ON A NUTRITIONAL RENAISSANCE

You'll also be celebrating the essence of nutrition. By valuing the origin, richness, and nourishing qualities of the foods you consume, you also foster a more fulfilling and balanced relationship with your meals. This holistic approach not only anchors your physical health but also nurtures your mental serenity during this transitional phase of life.

THE IMPORTANCE OF NUTRIENT-DENSE FOODS IN BLOOD SUGAR EQUILIBRIUM

One of the most important things that nutrient-dense foods do is to help regulate blood sugar levels. As you've learned in the previous chapter, this is important because when blood sugar is out of balance, it can make menopausal symptoms worse. Processed foods and sugary snacks might provide a quick energy fix, but they often lead to an inevitable crash, leaving you feeling lethargic and irritable.

In contrast, nutrient-dense foods ensure a steady, prolonged release of energy. By incorporating foods like whole grains, legumes, and avocados into the diet, you can achieve a more balanced blood sugar profile. This equilibrium is pivotal in reducing unexpected energy slumps and mood fluctuations, ensuring a more harmonious menopausal journey.

Moreover, maintaining stable blood sugar levels can also play a crucial role in metabolic health, supporting weight management and reducing the risk of conditions like insulin resistance. So, it's not just about feeling good in the moment, it's about setting the foundation for long-term wellness and vitality.

NUTRIENT-DENSE FOODS PROVIDE SYMPTOM RELIEF

The complexities of menopause demand that we pay better attention to what we choose to eat. This means not only selecting nutrient-dense foods to nourish the body but also those that specifically

CARA'S FAVORITE WAY TO . . .

Stop Cravings

Filling your plate with nourishing foods that make you feel full is far more rewarding than reaching for a tempting sugary donut. While the donut might offer a momentary treat, it often leaves you craving more. Instead, nourish your body first with a wholesome meal, rich in nutrients and designed to satisfy. Once you've enjoyed the lasting satiety it brings, you may find the pull of the donut has diminished. It's about feeding your body first with what it truly needs, and then deciding if you still have room for a sweet treat.

help to reduce the menopausal symptoms that can be problematic.

For example, phytoestrogens, naturally occurring chemical plant compounds in certain foods, like flaxseeds, can mimic the function of estrogen in the body. While they don't replace the hormone, they can offer some degree of symptom relief. Recognizing and integrating foods rich in these compounds can prove to be a game-changer, offering comfort amidst the ebb and flow of menopausal shifts. Let's learn more about them.

PHYTOESTROGENS: NATURE'S REMEDY TO EASE MENOPAUSAL SYMPTOMS

Phytoestrogens, the remarkable compounds found in various plants, play a unique role in mimicking the body's own estrogen, albeit with a lighter touch. They're not perfect matches for our estrogen, but their structural similarity enables them to interact gently with estrogen receptors. This interaction becomes particularly valuable during menopause, a time when natural estrogen levels are on a bit of a turbulent ride, eventually trending downward.

The beauty of phytoestrogens lies in their ability to ease some of the common discomforts associated with menopause. While they don't replace our natural estrogen, they act as a supportive buffer, helping to reduce symptoms. Essentially, phytoestrogens can be seen as a natural support system, offering a more comfortable and manageable transition through menopause. It's a wonderful example of how nature provides solutions that can help us navigate through life's changes with a bit more ease.

GLOBETROTTING INSIGHTS: THE POWER OF CULTURAL DIETS

There's compelling evidence from around the world that validates the potential of phytoestrogens. For instance, Asian cultures, particularly those in Japan, consume a diet rich in soy products, a potent source of phytoestrogens. Remarkably, numerous studies suggest that these women often experience fewer and less severe menopausal symptoms compared to their Western counterparts. Such observational insights provide a testament to the incredible impact diet can have on our overall physical condition.

In part 3, you'll find numerous recipes that incorporate and celebrate these sources of phyto-estrogens and other important nutrients. Not only do they provide potential relief from menopausal symptoms, but they also include a wide variety of flavors and textures, making each meal even more delicious.

By embracing phytoestrogens, you're not only adding a dietary component, you're also adopting a holistic approach that appreciates nature's wisdom, tapping into its reservoir of healing and balance.

Did You Know?

You can find phytoestrogens in a multitude of foods, including the following:

- **Soy and Soy Products:** Tofu, tempeh, and edamame

- **Seeds:** Flaxseeds and sesame seeds

- **Whole grains:** Oats, barley, and wheat bran

- **Legumes:** Lentils, chickpeas, and mung beans

- **Fruits:** Apples, carrots, and pomegranates

- **Vegetables:** Yams, broccoli, and alfalfa sprouts

Carbohydrates: Essential Energy for Menopausal Women

Over the past few decades, carbohydrates have been vilified in many diet trends, particularly those that promote high protein or fat consumption. This reputation stems from a simplified view of carbs, often lumping all carbohydrates into the "unhealthy" category. However, during menopause, the body undergoes hormonal shifts that can alter metabolism and energy levels. Carbohydrates, when chosen wisely, play a crucial role in supporting these changes.

SIMPLE VS. COMPLEX CARBOHYDRATES

Carbohydrates are the body's primary energy source. However, their structural differences dictate their impact on our health. Here's why:

1 **Simple Carbohydrates:** These are the basic sugars, easy for the body to break down. This might sound beneficial, but this rapid breakdown can lead to sudden peaks in blood sugar. Found in foods like cookies, cakes, white bread, and many processed foods, they often come with little nutritional value.

2 **Complex Carbohydrates:** Composed of longer chains of sugars, these molecules require more time for the body to digest. This means they provide a gradual, steady energy source. Rich in vitamins, minerals, and fibers, they're found in foods like oats, lentils, and broccoli.

THE HAZARDS OF OVERINDULGING IN SIMPLE CARBOHYDRATES

Reliance on simple carbs causes problems like the following:

1 **Volatile Blood Sugar Levels:** The quick absorption of these carbs causes sharp rises in blood sugar. This surge is usually followed by a drop, leading to an energy "crash," mood swings, and a sensation of hunger soon after eating.

2 **Insulin Resistance:** With recurrent highs and lows in blood sugar, the pancreas is prompted to produce insulin more frequently, raising the risk of insulin resistance over time. As we've seen, this is a condition where cells don't respond to insulin effectively, leading to elevated blood sugar levels.

3 **The Craving Cycle:** Simple carbs can trigger cravings. When blood sugar drops rapidly, the body craves quick energy, prompting desires for more sugary foods. Simultaneously, the stress of these fluctuations can result in elevated cortisol levels, exacerbating these cravings.

WHY COMPLEX CARBOHYDRATES ARE A BETTER CHOICE

Complex carbs provide many benefits, including the following:

1 **Stable Energy Reservoir:** The slow release of complex carbs ensures energy consistency, which is essential for maintaining focus and preventing fatigue throughout the day.

2 **Blood Sugar Equilibrium:** Complex carbs help maintain steady blood sugar levels, reducing the risk of type 2 diabetes and ensuring emotional and physical stability.

Small Steps, Big Results

Begin to add these ten complex carbohydrates to your diet for sustained energy, essential nutrients, and dietary fiber. When it comes to fiber, go slow to avoid gastrointestinal upset.

1	Whole grains	6	Oats
2	Legumes	7	Fiber-rich fruits
3	Starchy vegetables	8	Green vegetables
4	Whole grain breads	9	Whole grain cereals
5	Whole grain pastas	10	Nuts and seeds

So, you can see that while carbohydrates are essential, it's important to choose the right ones for health and wellness during menopause and beyond. Prioritize whole, unprocessed sources and be mindful of portion sizes. A rough guideline for menopausal women is to ensure their plates have about a quarter filled with wholesome carbs. This balance ensures adequate energy without overconsumption.

Carbohydrates, when understood and integrated wisely, can be powerful allies for menopausal women. They are not merely about energy but about holistic wellness, ensuring hormonal balance, emotional stability, and sustained vitality during this transformative phase of life.

Protein: The Nutritional Hero of Menopause

Proteins, crucial for nearly every bodily function, are large molecules composed of chains or building blocks of twenty different amino acids. The body is capable of synthesizing eleven of these amino acids; however, the remaining nine, known as "essential amino acids," must be obtained through our diet. These essential amino acids include histidine, isoleucine, leucine, lysine, methionine, phenylalanine, threonine, tryptophan, and valine.

Just as phytoestrogens play a key role during menopause by mimicking the body's estrogen to alleviate symptoms, amino acids are fundamental in constructing proteins that repair tissue, support immune function, and carry out numerous other critical tasks within the body. Ensuring a diet rich in essential amino acids is vital for maintaining health and supporting the body's myriad functions.

MENOPAUSE AND MUSCULAR CHANGE

When we age and especially during menopause, women face *sarcopenia*, which is the natural decline in muscle mass. This is exacerbated by hormonal changes, as declining estrogen levels can contribute to muscle loss. Muscle mass is not just about strength. It influences metabolism, bone density, and overall functionality.

WHY PROTEIN MATTERS SO MUCH IN MENOPAUSE

1 **Muscle Maintenance:** Consuming sufficient protein supports the maintenance of muscle mass. This is crucial during menopause, which is when we lose muscle faster.

2 **Enhanced Metabolism:** Muscle tissue requires more energy to maintain compared to fat tissue. By preserving or increasing muscle mass through protein intake and resistance exercises (more about this in part 2), postmenopausal women can combat the metabolic slowdown often experienced during this phase.

PROTEIN'S ROLE IN WEIGHT MANAGEMENT

Menopausal women often find managing weight a challenge. Protein is the friend you need. Here's why:

1 **Suppresses Appetite:** Protein plays a key role in regulating appetite by influencing hormones that control hunger and satiety. Specifically, consuming protein reduces the levels of ghrelin, often referred to as the "hunger hormone," which signals the brain to increase appetite.

At the same time, protein intake boosts the levels of peptide YY, a hormone that contributes to feelings of fullness. The decrease in ghrelin combined with the increase in peptide YY effectively helps to curb appetite, making you less likely to overeat and more likely to feel satisfied for longer periods after a meal. This dual effect makes protein an essential component of a weight management or healthy eating plan, as it assists in regulating energy intake by naturally moderating hunger signals.

2 **Thermic Effect of Food (TEF):** Protein has a higher TEF compared to fats and carbohydrates, meaning our body expends more energy (calories) to metabolize and store protein. This then aids in weight management. The higher TEF of protein results in an increased rate of calorie burn during digestion, making it a key nutrient for boosting metabolism and enhancing fat loss efforts.

Additionally, this energy-expanding process of digesting protein can contribute to a more efficient metabolic rate over time, increasing the body's ability to manage weight effectively. This makes protein an invaluable component of any diet focused on healthy weight management or loss.

3 **Bone Health and Protein:** The conversation around bones often centers on calcium and vitamin D, but protein's role is equally paramount. Protein makes up about 50 percent of bone volume and about one-third of bone mass. A diet rich in protein, when combined with adequate calcium intake, supports bone density, reducing the risk of fractures and osteoporosis in postmenopausal women.

4 **Deciphering Protein Needs:** While generic guidelines suggest 1.2 grams of protein per kilogram (2.2 pounds) of body weight for menopausal women, it's essential to understand that individual needs can vary. Factors influencing protein requirements include activity level, muscle mass, overall health, and specific health goals.

PROTEIN: WHY VARIETY MATTERS

A varied protein intake ensures a spectrum of amino acids and other accompanying nutrients, promoting a well-rounded nutritional profile that supports overall health. Let's take a closer look.

1 **Animal-Derived Proteins:** Fish, especially fatty ones like salmon, mackerel, anchovies, sardines, and herring (think SMASH), all contain omega-3 fatty acids. Poultry, preferably lean cuts like chicken breasts, provides protein without much saturated fat. Eggs, especially egg whites, are protein powerhouses.

2 **Plant-Based Protein:** Quinoa is a rare plant food that provides all nine essential amino acids. Lentils, apart from being protein-rich, also offer dietary fiber. Edamame and tofu, both derived from soybeans, are complete protein sources, and they bring along isoflavones, which might help with certain menopausal symptoms. A shift toward plant-based proteins can also reduce water usage, greenhouse gas emissions, and land use, which means you're committed to a more environmentally sustainable diet.

THE BENEFITS OF PLANT PROTEINS

Opting for plant-derived proteins offers a host of benefits that extends well beyond just providing essential amino acids. These benefits play a significant role in various aspects of health, including digestive health and heart health.

1 **Digestive Health:** The inclusion of plant-based proteins in your diet is beneficial for digestive health due to the high fiber content found in these sources. Foods such as legumes, nuts, and seeds not only supply protein but also a significant amount of dietary fiber, which is crucial for maintaining a healthy gut.

Fiber helps to regulate bowel movements, prevent constipation, and reduce the risk of digestive disorders. Additionally, the fiber in plant-based protein sources acts as a prebiotic, feeding the beneficial bacteria in the gut and thus promoting a balanced and healthy microbiome. This, in turn, can enhance nutrient absorption and strengthen the immune system.

2 **Heart Health:** When it comes to heart health, plant proteins offer several protective benefits. Many plant-based sources of protein, such as beans, lentils, and tofu, are naturally low in saturated fat and cholesterol-free, contributing to lower cholesterol levels and improved lipid profiles.

These foods also often contain heart-healthy nutrients like fiber, omega-3 fatty acids, and antioxidants, which can help reduce inflammation and lower blood pressure. Regular consumption of plant proteins has been linked to a reduced risk of developing heart disease, stroke, and hypertension, making them a smart choice for anyone looking to support their cardiovascular health.

Incorporating a variety of plant-based proteins into your diet not only diversifies your nutrient intake but also leverages these health benefits, contributing to a healthful life and chronic disease prevention.

Fiber: The Unsung Hero of Menopausal Nutrition

At the heart of a balanced menopausal diet is fiber, a component often overshadowed by the more widely discussed macronutrients like proteins and carbohydrates. However, for menopausal women, understanding and embracing the significance of fiber can lead to many health benefits, particularly in the context of weight maintenance.

WHAT IS FIBER?

Fiber is a type of complex carbohydrate found in all plant-based foods that travels through our digestive system largely unchanged. It stands out because unlike proteins, fats, and simple carbohydrates, it doesn't break down to provide energy directly. Instead, fiber's significance lies in its comprehensive benefits for digestive health, weight management, and overall well-being, making it an indispensable part of a healthy diet.

FIBER'S ROLE IN DIGESTIVE HEALTH

Digestion is a complex journey, and fiber is a crucial navigator along this path, especially in the small and large intestines.

1 **Small Intestine:** In the small intestine, where the breakdown of food occurs and nutrients are absorbed, fiber plays a crucial role. It slows the absorption of sugars, preventing those sharp increases in blood sugar levels. This slow-release mechanism provided by fiber ensures a more consistent and sustained energy level, avoiding the rapid spikes that can lead to energy crashes.

2 **Large Intestine:** The large intestine's primary functions include water and electrolyte absorption and the transformation of waste into stool. Fiber significantly contributes to this process by adding bulk to the stool, facilitating its passage and preventing issues like constipation. This bulkiness also speeds up the movement of food and waste, helping to maintain a healthy digestive tract.

CARA'S FAVORITE
WAY TO . . .
Eat Less Without Counting Calories

Incorporating plant-based proteins into your diet can be a strategic move, particularly if you're focusing on weight management. Typically, plant proteins are lower in calories compared to their meat counterparts, offering a double benefit: They not only contribute to your protein intake but can also help in eating less calories. So, even if you enjoy meat, diversifying your protein sources with plants can be a flavorful and helpful way to support your weight loss goals.

THE CONNECTION BETWEEN FIBER AND WEIGHT MAINTENANCE

For individuals, particularly menopausal women, aiming to maintain a stable weight, fiber offers several advantages:

1 **Satiety and Fullness:** Foods high in fiber tend to be more satisfying, which can lead to a natural reduction in calorie intake. Feeling fuller for longer periods helps to curb the urge to snack and overeat, aiding in weight management efforts.

2 **Stabilized Blood Sugar:** Fiber's ability to moderate blood sugar spikes plays a key role in maintaining energy levels and preventing hunger that can lead to overeating. This steadiness helps in managing cravings and supports a balanced diet.

3 Fiber Improves Gut Health: Beyond digestion, fiber nourishes the beneficial bacteria in our gut. A thriving microbiome is associated with better metabolic health, reduced inflammation, and even positive mood regulation. For menopausal women, a balanced gut can help in managing some of the common symptoms of menopause such as brain fog and mood swings.

DIETARY SOURCES OF FIBER

Nature generously provides a wide range of fiber-rich foods that are essential for our health. Fruits and vegetables are key contributors, offering soluble fiber that helps in regulating blood sugar levels and lowering cholesterol. They also supply insoluble fiber, crucial for maintaining digestive health and preventing constipation.

Whole grains are another important source, delivering both types of fiber along with essential nutrients that bolster health and vitality. Legumes are notable for their high fiber and protein content, making them a significant part of a balanced diet. By including a variety of these foods in your daily intake, you can support gut health, manage weight effectively, and decrease the risk of chronic diseases, which reinforces the importance of fiber in a healthy lifestyle. Make sure to add fiber-rich foods slowly as they may cause gastrointestinal upset.

GOOD FIBER SOURCES

- **Fruits:** Apples, berries, pears, and oranges
- **Vegetables:** Broccoli, brussels sprouts, and carrots
- **Legumes:** Lentils, black beans, and chickpeas
- **Whole Grains:** Quinoa, barley, and oats
- **Seeds:** Chia seeds and flaxseeds

THE SYNERGY BETWEEN FIBER AND MENOPAUSE

Menopause marks a significant period of transition in a woman's life, bringing about various physical and hormonal changes. In this transformative phase, the nutritional roles of carbohydrates, proteins, and fats are well-acknowledged, yet the critical importance of dietary fiber is often minimized.

HOW TO . . .
Feel Full Longer

Eating a combination of protein, fiber, and carbohydrates is an effective nutritional strategy because these nutrients work synergistically to support overall health and stabilize blood sugar levels. Protein is essential for building and repairing tissues, and it promotes satiety, helping to reduce overall calorie intake.

Fiber, especially the types found in whole grains, vegetables, and fruits, aids in digestion and slows the absorption of sugars into the bloodstream, preventing spikes in blood sugar levels. This slow release of glucose provides a more consistent energy supply. Including carbohydrates, particularly complex ones like those in whole grains and starchy vegetables, is crucial as they are the body's primary energy source.

Together, these nutrients ensure a balanced diet, providing sustained energy, aiding in weight management, and supporting metabolic health, making them particularly beneficial in a diet aimed at maintaining steady blood sugar levels.

Fiber's role extends far beyond just aiding digestion. It becomes a cornerstone of health, particularly for menopausal women. Its benefits are multifaceted, including enhancing digestive wellness, which is crucial as the body adapts to hormonal fluctuations. Additionally, fiber plays a pivotal role in weight management, a common concern during menopause, by promoting feelings of fullness and reducing overall calorie intake.

Moreover, fiber contributes to stabilizing blood sugar levels and may help in lowering the risk of heart disease by reducing cholesterol levels. This synergy between fiber intake and menopause management underscores the value of incorporating a fiber-rich diet to navigate this natural life stage with greater ease and health.

In part 3, you'll find recipes rich in fiber to make it easier to seamlessly add this vital nutrient into your daily meals.

Why Gut Health Matters in Menopause: More Than Just Digestion

Finally, it's important to understand the gut and how it affects the body and mind. Our gut, often dubbed our "second brain," plays a pivotal role beyond digestion, significantly influencing our health, emotions, and well-being, particularly during menopause. This complex interplay between our gut and brain is facilitated by the vagus nerve, a key component of the parasympathetic nervous system responsible for "rest and digest" functions.

STIMULATING THE VAGUS NERVE

Extending from the brain to the abdomen, the vagus nerve serves as a bi-directional communication highway, affecting mood, stress levels, and mental clarity. Stimulating this nerve through practices like deep breathing exercises can enhance relaxation and mental stability. It creates a bridge between our physiological states and emotional health. Slow, deep inhalations followed by extended exhalations stimulate the vagus nerve, help the gut-brain axis stay in balance, and even reduce inflammation. You'll find a meditation designed to specifically soothe the vagus nerve in chapter 6.

KEEPING THE MICROBIOME HEALTHY

It's also important to know that our gut hosts a vast universe of microorganisms, known as the *microbiome*, comprising bacteria, viruses, and fungi. A healthy microbiome, characterized by a balance of beneficial and harmful bacteria, is crucial for digestion, nutrient absorption, and immune function.

Disruptions in this balance can lead to a host of issues, underscoring the importance of dietary choices in cultivating a healthy gut environment. Foods rich in fiber, along with fermented products like yogurt and sauerkraut, nourish beneficial bacteria, while limiting sugar and processed foods helps prevent the proliferation of harmful bacteria.

THE GUT-BRAIN AXIS: WHY IT MATTERS

The gut-brain axis represents a dynamic two-way street, with constant communication that influences our emotions, appetite, and decision-making. Remarkably, over 90 percent of serotonin, a neurotransmitter linked to mood, is produced in the gut, which shows how important a balanced microbiome is to our emotional health. For menopausal women, who may experience mood swings and emotional challenges due to hormonal fluctuations, maintaining gut health can provide emotional stability and resilience.

Focusing on gut health during menopause is not just about supporting digestion but fostering overall health and emotional balance. With hormones in flux, a resilient gut can enhance energy levels, stabilize mood, and improve sleep quality. The rapidly increasing field of gut health research underscores the importance of nurturing our gut as a means of nurturing our entire being.

By embracing practical strategies, dietary adjustments, and lifestyle changes aimed at improving gut health, we can navigate menopause gracefully and lay the groundwork for lasting health and vitality. This holistic approach not only addresses the challenges of menopause but also enriches our overall quality of life, demonstrating the critical role of gut health in our journey toward wellness.

In the next chapter, we'll examine another pivotal aspect of our menopausal journey: exercise. Menopause invokes unique challenges and demands, so it's absolutely necessary to change your approach to physical activity. I'll show you how to do just that.

Action Steps

Keep in mind that awareness is the key to making positive changes. Try these Action Steps to help you make better choices when it comes to what you're eating and to get rid of the habits that are not serving you well.

1 **Write down your pain points** with regard to food and drink. Where do you struggle? These are the things that you always stumble at, what holds you back, your triggers, or what stops you from starting. Is it that 11 a.m. snack or the first glass of wine at night that leads to another two or three? Mindless eating in front of the TV? Or not knowing when to stop when you are full?

2 **How do your pain points trigger** you to eat or drink when you'd rather not?

3 **Work to avoid your triggers.** Move your breakfast an hour later to stop the 11 a.m. munchies. Go for a walk at the time the wine bottle calls. Go to bed an hour earlier so you are not tempted to snack at night. Fill your plate with veggies and have as much as you'd like.

4 **Try breathing techniques** when a craving calls. My go-to easy breath technique is *box breathing*. Here's how to do it: Breathe in for a count of four, hold for a count of four, breathe out for four counts, and hold for four counts. Repeat this for three minutes or until you feel the craving subside. When your mind wonders, just come back to focusing on your breath. Wandering thoughts are normal. Do not fight them. It takes time to change habits though, so don't expect to be a master right away!

5 **Have a large glass of water** when you feel hungry, wait ten minutes, and then see if you still feel hungry.

6 **When you feel hungry** for high sugar or simple carbohydrates, ask yourself if you could eat a whole plate of broccoli. If the answer is no, then you are not that hungry! Your mind is a powerful thing. Learn to master the cravings so they don't control you.

7 **Become more mindful** of your pain points and triggers and practice the strategies that work for you until they become a habit. This will help you to stop eating the wrong foods and begin eating the right ones to ease your menopausal symptoms.

6

The Change Means Changing Your Workouts

Reaching forty is not just a milestone age but also a turning point for your body. As you navigate through this new chapter of life, it's essential to recognize that the exercise regimen that served you well in your twenties and thirties might not be as effective or suitable now. Let's delve into understanding why the dynamics of exercise shift after forty and how you can tailor your workouts to match your body's evolving needs.

Hormonal Shifts: Navigating Life's Changes

As you move through menopause and beyond, it's crucial to acknowledge and understand the symphony of hormonal changes playing in the background. These shifts aren't just internal alterations. They influence your physical vitality, emotional balance, and overall well-being. Let's take another look at these hormones, how menopausal changes affect the jobs they do, and how this impacts fitness.

ESTROGEN'S MULTIFACETED ROLE

One of the cornerstones of female health, estrogen isn't merely a reproductive hormone. It plays a vital role in preserving bone density, ensuring skin elasticity, and regulating the body's energy use, fat storage, and even insulin production. As estrogen levels decline, you'll probably notice changes in weight, particularly around the abdomen, accelerated bone loss, leading to conditions like osteoporosis, and mood fluctuations.

PROGESTERONE'S BALANCING ACT

Progesterone harmoniously pairs with estrogen to orchestrate several bodily functions. Its decline might lead to irregular menstrual cycles, noticeable mood variations, and for some, bouts of insomnia. Together, estrogen and progesterone jointly maintain bone vitality. Lower levels can speed up bone density loss, causing bones to become fragile and more prone to fractures.

TESTOSTERONE: NOT JUST FOR MEN

While testosterone is often associated with males, it's pivotal for women too. Testosterone is responsible for building muscle, fat metabolism, and maintaining libido, so a decrease in testosterone can lead to an increase in body fat, a decrease in sexual desire, and diminishing muscle mass. A decrease in muscle doesn't only signify reduced strength, but also a slowing metabolism, posing challenges in calorie burning and potential weight gain.

INSULIN RESISTANCE AND EXERCISE

Overall, the intricate dance of hormones during this time can lead to a more lethargic metabolism. As we've seen, insulin resistance occurs when cells in the body become less responsive to insulin, a hormone produced by the pancreas that allows cells to absorb glucose and convert it into energy. This resistance can be exacerbated by hormonal imbalances, particularly during periods of significant change such as menopause, when fluctuating hormone levels can impact the body's sensitivity to insulin.

With increased insulin resistance, the body finds it challenging to efficiently convert sugars to energy, leading to fat storage instead of being used as a fuel source. This process not only contributes to weight gain but also strains the body's metabolic health, highlighting the importance of managing insulin sensitivity through diet, exercise, and lifestyle modifications.

Armed with this understanding, it becomes evident that your exercise regimen during menopause needs an overhaul. The focus needs to shift from working out *harder* to working out *smarter*. Part of this process is to recognize that bone density and joint flexibility change in menopause and how to counteract it.

Bone Density and Joint Health: How They Affect Fitness

The telltale signs of aging don't just manifest on the skin. Beneath the surface, there are many changes happening, especially concerning your bone density and joint health. As you journey into menopause, there's a natural decline in bone mass. As we've seen, this decline can increase the risk of osteoporosis and fractures. Your joints, having served you loyally over the years, may become less flexible and you might experience occasional aches and pains you never felt before.

This isn't meant to sound an alarm but to raise awareness. With the right exercise regimen, you can not only reduce these risks but also potentially reverse some of the early signs. You'll find a variety of exercises to do just this in part 2, but first, let's learn a bit about the different ways you can improve joint flexibility and balance, build better bones, and more.

IMPROVING JOINT FLEXIBILITY

Remember those joint aches or stiffness you occasionally feel after a long day? They're your joints' way of reminding you to show them some love. So, it's important to incorporate exercises that promote joint flexibility. Think dynamic stretches, mobility drills, and even dance. And while we're on the topic of gentle exercise, don't forget the magic of yoga. Those stretches and poses aren't just good for the soul. They're great for joint health.

PRIORITIZING BALANCE

With declining bone density and joint flexibility, it's crucial to work on balance exercises. Improving your stability can prevent falls and subsequent fractures. Incorporate routines that challenge and improve your balance, even if it's as simple as standing on one foot for a few seconds every day. Yoga poses like the mountain, tree, and triangle are also helpful when it comes to improving your balance.

STRENGTH TRAINING: BONES' BEST FRIEND

When it comes to enhancing bone density, strength training is gold. Every time you engage in weight-bearing exercises, you're essentially sending a signal to your body to bolster bone formation. This doesn't mean you need to become a professional weightlifter overnight. Simple resistance exercises, tailored to your comfort and capability, can make a substantial difference.

The beauty of strength training lies not only in its ability to sculpt and tone but in the profound benefits it provides, particularly as the years roll by. Many perceive strength training as the domain of the young and the athletic. Still, its advantages become even more pronounced and crucial as you mature. One of the most important benefits of strength training is that it preserves muscle mass and revs up your metabolism.

PRESERVING MUSCLE MASS
AND BOOSTING METABOLISM

It's an inescapable fact of biology that as the years progress, the muscle mass that once came so effortlessly in youth begins to wane. This decline can commence as early as your thirties and accelerates with each passing decade. What's the side effect? You have a metabolism that's slower and less responsive. This can manifest as weight gain, reduced strength, and a lack of energy.

Strength training can help by regularly challenging your muscles with resistance, whether from weights, resistance bands, or your body weight, by sending a clear call to your body to repair and rebuild. What's the result? You not only maintain but can even grow muscle mass. And with more muscle, you keep the metabolic fires burning

brighter and longer. It's your secret weapon against the sluggish metabolic tendencies of aging.

BUILDING BONE DENSITY:
YOUR DEFENSE AGAINST OSTEOPOROSIS

Just as muscles respond to resistance, so do your bones. Think of strength training as a conversation you're having with your skeletal system. Each squat, deadlift, or resistance exercise tells your bones, "You need to be strong, resilient, and ready for anything."

In response, bones undergo a process called *bone remodeling*, where old bone tissue is replaced with new bone. Strength training stimulates this process, encouraging increased bone density. This proactive approach is vital in fending off osteoporosis—a condition that makes bones fragile and more prone to fractures. Regular weight-bearing exercises can serve as both prevention and remedy, ensuring that your skeletal foundation remains robust and steadfast.

To truly optimize the benefits of strength training, it's essential to adopt a holistic view. This means not only focusing on the exercises themselves but ensuring proper technique, incorporating adequate rest, and pairing your efforts with nutrition that

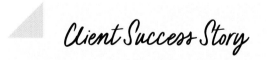

Client Success Story

Cara's plan has totally transformed my shape, weight, strength, and fitness levels. I've done this by committing without fail to a fifteen-minute workout for at least five days a week. My family has been amazed at the changes.   **—LINDA**

fuels muscle growth and recovery. In part 2, you'll learn how to adopt an effective strength training routine tailored to your unique needs to help you move through this transformative phase of life.

Time to Rethink Cardio

You've seen the benefits of strength training when it comes to building bone density and improving flexibility. As we age, cardiovascular exercise should also be in your fitness mix. The rhythmic pounding of feet on the pavement, the exhilarating rush of a high-intensity interval training session, or the simple joy of a brisk walk in the park—cardio has long been a favorite in the fitness realm.

From burning calories to enhancing mood, it promises many benefits. But as you transition through menopause, a stage marked by hormonal shifts and new physiological challenges, it's essential to reconsider the role of cardiovascular workouts in your routine.

THE CARDIO MYTH: BEYOND THE HEARTBEAT

Yes, cardiovascular exercises are instrumental in promoting heart health. Every elevated heartbeat speaks to improved circulation, lung capacity, and enhanced cardiovascular stamina. However, a prevailing notion suggests that "more is always better," a concept that needs reevaluation, especially during menopause.

Intensive, high-impact cardio, when overdone, can be counterproductive. While pushing the limits can sometimes feel empowering, excessive stress on the body can lead to burnout. Overtraining doesn't just fatigue muscles. It can strain the heart and the very system you're trying to strengthen. Furthermore, it can disrupt hormonal balance, contributing to irregularities that affect overall well-being, underscoring the need for moderation

and rest in any fitness regimen to promote health rather than compromise it.

With the hormonal changes of menopause, particularly the decline in estrogen, high-intensity workouts can elevate cortisol levels, our primary stress hormone. Chronic high levels of cortisol, especially during menopause, can exacerbate symptoms like sleep disturbances and mood swings, and can also lead to increased abdominal fat. Additionally, this imbalance in cortisol may hinder the body's ability to recover effectively from exercise, reducing the benefits of physical activity and potentially impacting long-term health and fitness goals.

BALANCED CARDIO: THE MIDDLE PATH

This isn't a call to abandon cardio. It's a reminder to find a harmonious balance. As you navigate menopause, moderation and mindfulness become paramount. Choosing moderate-intensity workouts, such as a serene walk, a steady bike ride, or a dance class, can offer cardiovascular advantages without the potential cortisol surge. Such exercises become particularly valuable when managing menopausal symptoms, helping to alleviate mood fluctuations and improve life quality.

Tuning into your body's signals becomes even more crucial during this period. Post-workout, if you're left feeling rejuvenated and spirited, you're on the right path. However, if lingering fatigue, discomfort, or pain overshadows the afterglow, it might be time to reassess.

As you venture through menopause, exercise becomes a balancing act. Cardio, while essential, plays a more nuanced role. It intertwines with strength training, tranquility exercises, and meditation to forge a comprehensive health blueprint, tailored to meet the unique demands of this transitional life phase. We'll look at the importance of meditation next.

Small Steps, Big Results

I personally no longer feel the need for long workouts because I get results in a quarter of the time I spent exercising before! Let's face it, long workouts are not always sustainable with a busy lifestyle. But short workouts allow you to stay consistent. My clients have found that consistency is key to results, not stopping and starting with exercise and diet regimes.

Meditation: A Vital Component of Your Fitness Routine

Without a doubt, physical activity lays the foundation for a robust body. It builds bone density and improves flexibility, muscle tone, and heart health. But what about the epicenter of our being, the mind?

As you transition into and through menopause, the fitness narrative undergoes a profound transformation. The focus expands beyond muscle toning and cardiovascular endurance into the realm of mental resilience and emotional equilibrium. It's not just about the heart's beats but also the mind's beats. Here, the gentle art of meditation, a serene dance of the soul, emerges as an incredible tool in your workout library.

HORMONAL HARMONY: FINDING BALANCE IN THE MIDDLE OF THE CHAOS

The menopausal journey, with its ebb and flow of hormones, is like navigating a sea with both calm waters and sudden storms. Hormonal fluctuations can cause mood swings, foggy thinking, and even bouts of anxiety.

Estrogen and progesterone levels go down, but stress, if unchecked, can cause cortisol (as we've seen, this is a hormone closely associated with stress) to surge. Elevated cortisol levels not only accentuate some menopausal symptoms but can also disrupt the delicate hormonal harmony.

Meditation acts as an anchor in these turbulent times, helping you to manage stress, which in turn helps to balance cortisol levels. A meditation practice also carves out a space for reflection, enhances mental clarity, sharpens focus, and fosters emotional balance. It's like strength training but for the mind, as you build resilience to handle the mental and emotional upheavals that menopause (and life) can sometimes throw your way.

This restorative practice offers more than just momentary calm. It bolsters a harmonious hormonal environment, which is paramount during menopause. Through focused breathing, mindfulness, and grounding techniques, meditation promotes an inner equilibrium, ensuring that amidst the hormonal shifts, there remains a center of stability.

As menopause unfolds, remember that your holistic wellness encompasses both body and mind. Meditation, though seemingly passive, is an active measure to bolster your mental and emotional state. You'll find three meditation practices here and the resources to find many more.

NEW TO MEDITATION? TRY THIS.

This simple practice can be a powerful tool to calm the mind and relax the body. Remember, meditation is a skill that develops with practice, so be patient and kind to yourself as you learn.

- Choose a calm and quiet place where you won't be disturbed.

- Sit or lie down in a comfortable position. You can use a chair, a cushion, or even your bed. The key is to keep your back straight to maintain alertness.

- Close your eyes to reduce visual distractions.

- Focus on your breath. Notice the sensation of air entering and leaving your nostrils or the rise and fall of your chest. You don't need to change your breathing pattern, just observe it.

- When your mind wanders (and it will), gently acknowledge the thoughts without judgment and bring your focus back to your breath. This practice of returning to the breath builds mindfulness.

Menopause 101: Ease Stress and More with Exercise and Meditation

Learning to manage your stress through exercise and meditation is an effective way to control your weight and avoid belly fat. When we relax, the body doesn't need to pump out cortisol, so the adrenal glands can focus on producing estrogen to help balance your hormonal levels. This means your body won't need to depend on the cells in belly fat to produce estrogen to make up the gap. Learning stress-busting techniques is vital for you to learn if you want to control your weight during menopause.

- If you're just starting, aim for a short duration, like five minutes. You can gradually increase the time as you get more comfortable with the practice.

- When your time ends, slowly open your eyes. Take a moment to notice how your body feels and the state of your mind. Then, gently transition back to your day.

MEDITATION FOR THE VAGUS NERVE DURING MENOPAUSE

The vagus nerve is a key part of our parasympathetic nervous system, running from the brainstem through the body to various organs. This "rest and digest" nerve helps control heart rate, digestion, and mood, and is essential for reducing stress and inflammation. This meditation that stimulates the vagus nerve nurtures your body, soothes your nervous system, and promotes a sense of calmness and peacefulness. Here's how to do it:

- Find a quiet place where you won't be disturbed. Sit in a comfortable position, either on a chair with your feet flat on the ground, cross-legged on a cushion, or lie down, whichever feels best for you.

- Inhale slowly (four seconds): Gently inhale through your nose, counting to four. Fill your lungs, expand your diaphragm, and welcome calmness into your body.

- Hold (seven seconds): Hold your breath for a count of seven, allowing stillness to spread throughout your body.

- Exhale gradually (eight seconds): Exhale slowly through your mouth for eight counts, releasing tension, stress, or discomfort.

- Pause (two seconds): After exhaling, pause briefly in the quiet space before the next breath, feeling the relief of letting go.

- Repeat: Continue this breathing pattern for ten minutes. With each cycle, imagine deepening your body's relaxation, calming your mind, and enriching your spirit with peace.

- As you breathe, envision your breath as a gentle wave, massaging and stimulating your vagus nerve. This visualization can enhance the nerve's tone, promoting a state of calm throughout your body and mind.

- Gradually return to the present, moving your fingers and toes, and gently stretch. Open your eyes when ready and bring the tranquility and balance from this session into your day.

RESOURCES FOR LEARNING TO MEDITATE

- **ZenMe App:** This is an incredible app by Camilla Sacre-Dallerup. It contains meditations and courses for self-development and peace.

- **Unplug:** The Unplug Meditation app has the largest collection of practical meditations to help you overcome life's obstacles and get things done.

- **Insight Timer:** This is a free app with thousands of guided meditations from practitioners around the world on various subjects.

Shifting Your Approach to Exercise and Wellness

The journey through menopause and life after forty is a transformative time, not just hormonally, but physically and mentally as well. As the tides of time shift, so too should our approach to wellness.

Embracing the power of strength training becomes paramount to counteract the natural decline in muscle mass and bone density, while improving joint flexibility and balance enables us to live active lives. Instead of becoming a frail, old woman, you'll be strong, vibrant, and full of life and able to cope with all that our later years will throw at us.

While the benefits of cardiovascular exercise remain undeniable, a revised and balanced cardio routine ensures you reap the rewards without inadvertently elevating levels of the stress hormone cortisol.

But it's not just about the weights you lift or the miles you run. It's also important to nurture peace and serenity during this turbulent time. A regular meditation practice ensures mental agility and emotional resilience during hormonal ebbs and flows.

In essence, adapting to life during and after menopause is about embracing a holistic philosophy. It's about intertwining the strength of the body with the resilience of the mind. By integrating diverse exercises with the restorative powers of meditation, you cultivate a regimen that's attuned to your evolving needs.

This harmonized approach promises not just physical energy but also mental clarity and emotional serenity. As you navigate this unique chapter of life, remember that it's about forging a path that resonates with every facet of your being, ensuring a mix of vitality, strength, and peace.

Action Steps

1 **Look ahead to part 2** and familiarize yourself with the workout schedule. Decide when you'll start your 4-Week, 15-Minute Plan.

2 **Schedule the days and times** you'll work out, meditate, or walk.

3 **If you feel overwhelmed** or daunted, just remind yourself that *you can do this*! You can do it one day, one workout, one meditation session, or one walk at a time. You deserve to find *you* again.

4 **Read the next chapter** to help you achieve and maintain the positive mindset that you need to complete the plan.

7

Why a Positive Mindset Is Everything

Menopause marks not just a biological transition, but a chance to reshape our approach to health and happiness. In this chapter, I'll guide you through setting realistic goals—think of them as your personal markers of success—easily within grasp rather than frustratingly beyond reach.

The 80/20 Rule

Following the 80/20 rule changes everything. Let me explain what this rule is and why it works. 80 percent of the time, you engage in behaviors that deeply nourish and benefit you, from eating wholesome foods to enjoying enriching activities and restful sleep. What about the remaining 20 percent? That's your built-in flexibility, the space that allows for life's unpredictability and the occasional indulgence. This is not about stringent adherence to a strict regimen, but rather about finding a harmonious balance that accommodates the natural ebb and flow of life.

You'll focus on the concept of addition rather than subtraction, emphasizing the power of incorporating beneficial practices and nutrient-rich foods into your daily routine. This approach helps to organically phase out less healthy habits without the sense of loss and restriction that often comes with traditional diets. The goal is to adopt a lifestyle that ends the cycle of yo-yo dieting and sets the stage for a stable, fulfilling way of living where wellness is your natural state.

Remember that this journey is about progressive evolution, not immediate transformation. It's about the small, intentional steps that lead to monumental changes over time, which is what you'll learn about next, along with setting goals, building confidence, making time for self-care, and getting clear about what you hope to achieve and why. After that, we'll circle back to the 80/20 rule, and you'll learn how to put it into practice.

Get ready to embrace a new mindset where every small positive choice is a victory and every day is an opportunity to thrive.

Does this sound good to you?

Let's get to it!

Embrace the Gentle Ascent: Small Goals, Big Impact

When it comes to the journey of personal health and well-being, especially as we navigate the unpredictable time of menopause, the power of setting small, attainable goals cannot be overstated. This strategy, which is similar to preparing for a series of gentle hills rather than a single daunting mountain, emphasizes progress through patience and persistence. By focusing on achievable steps, we allow ourselves the grace to adapt and the strength to persevere, making the journey not only manageable but deeply rewarding.

THE POWER OF MODEST PROMISES

Setting big goals can be a setup for failure. They often seem too large, feel too daunting, and can lead to sensory overload, which stops progress before it even begins. Conversely, smaller goals are like stepping stones across a stream: manageable, achievable, and they keep you moving forward. These modest promises you make to yourself are fundamental. They build a bridge of trust and self-confidence. Each time you take a small step, you are reinforcing your belief in your ability to succeed.

HABIT FORMATION: THE BEDROCK OF LASTING CHANGE

When you hold yourself to these gentle commitments, you're not only more likely to maintain consistency, but you're also crafting a habit, a routine that becomes second nature, a thread woven seamlessly into the fabric of your life. This habit formation is the bedrock of true, lasting change, not the short-lived results born from spurts of deprivation and discipline.

HOW TO . . .

Keep the Promises You Make to Yourself

Creating and meeting personal commitments is a powerful way to build inner confidence. Consider the unease you'd feel if you neglected to prepare for a crucial speech or exam. It's a similar sentiment when you don't prioritize self-care. Treat the promises you make for your own well-being as non-negotiable appointments. Commit to actions that nurture and respect your body. This dedication will cultivate a profound and steadfast confidence from within.

Start with small, manageable promises to yourself today. Watch as this self-assurance transforms your approach to life's challenges and feel your confidence grow.

For example, if you promise that you'll do a fifteen-minute workout at 7 a.m. tomorrow and you do it, the feeling of empowerment is incredible. Or if you promise yourself that in your lunch break, you'll go for a brisk walk for twenty minutes and you do, then you'll have a sense of achievement. All this moves you to the inner confidence I want for you.

MAKE SELF-CARE A PRIORITY

In the tapestry of life, menopause is a period often marked by the demands of family, career, and personal upheaval. Often, time for self-care can seem scarce. That's precisely why these small, daily goals are vital. They are the commitments that fit into your life, rather than the ones that demand you reshape your life around them. They are the non-negotiables that deserve your time and your energy, affirming that self-care is not only necessary but essential.

ROUTINE IS YOUR FRIEND

Routine is everything. All the time you are sporadic with your efforts, you'll never see the results that you are striving for. Creating habits, routine, and discipline is where you need to focus. In embracing this approach, you're not merely surviving this stage of life, you're thriving.

You're learning that the art of keeping a promise to yourself is as crucial as it is to others. This creates a feeling of strength beyond the physical and resilience that is renewing. It's in the everyday dedication to these small acts of self-care that the incredible results you crave begin to happen, creating a lifestyle of wellness that's as sustainable as it is satisfying.

SET YOURSELF UP FOR SUCCESS: POWER OF WRITTEN GOALS

Writing down your goals is a simple but powerful act that anchors your intentions in the real world. When you do this, your goals transition from thoughts in your head to tangible targets.

ENVISIONING THE FUTURE: LONG-TERM GOALS

Write down the main goal that you want to achieve. Don't be shy or embarrassed about what you want. Only you know what the driver of your goals is. Have that vision and see it clearly. Start by defining your ultimate destination. Dreams or goals will guide your path. For me, it's to live in a happy and healthy old age.

WHY MID-TERM GOALS MATTER TOO

I often also focus on mid-term goals. This means focusing on something that's not too far off and enables me to work toward it and see the results sooner. As I write this book, my mid-term goal is to feel as confident and healthy as I can when my eldest daughter gets married. This pushes me to focus even more closely on my diet, exercise, and mind-body-spirit nourishment.

I encourage you to find a mid-term goal you can focus on, maybe a vacation or trip or an anniversary or birthday celebration, as you journey toward the life you want to create.

Identify the significant milestones you wish to reach. Whether it's improving your health and your weight or looking your best for a special occasion you have coming up, these goals act as a light guiding your journey.

MEETING GOALS MEANS TAKING DAILY STEPS TO ACHIEVE THEM

No matter what your goal may be—mid-term or long-term—the most important thing to keep in mind is that it takes steps to get there. Focus on the week ahead and divide each goal into short-term manageable actions. When you take these daily steps on a consistent basis, it will construct the staircase to your ultimate goal. A step can be as simple as adding more water to your daily intake, taking a walk each day, starting to meditate, or adding a new nutritious food to your diet.

MOVE FORWARD BUT FOCUS ON THE NOW

As you move forward, focus on the *now*, not what lies ahead. Take one day at a time and know that each day is a step toward where you want to be. This is important. Once your goals are set, always return your focus to the present. While your long-term and mid-term goals provide direction, dwelling on them can be overwhelming. Direct your energy to fulfilling your short-term promises that you have set yourself each day.

THE DAILY TRIUMPHS:
NON-NEGOTIABLE SMALL WINS

Celebrating each small win is such a powerful tool. So many times, we are hard on ourselves for what we didn't do and forget the things we did do! Celebrate each win with a smile and realize how you are winning at this thing called *life*!

Small Steps, Big Results

Once you believe in this process, the magic of results will happen. When you only focus on big goals, you never seem to get there, and if you do reach your goals, it's not as satisfying. When the process is just too diffi- cult, it makes it hard to feel good and makes it easier to give up. Often old habits creep back in and before you know it, you're back where you started and then some.

Adopt the philosophy of the compound effect. Just as small financial investments grow over time, so too do the little daily efforts that grow into significant life changes and lead to a lifestyle of complete- ness and contentment. For example, not buying that pack of cookies because you tell yourself that your partner will love to have them but then eating them yourself on the way home in the car (this is me!).

Commit to small, daily objectives that are non- negotiable. Each fulfilled promise, no matter how minor, is a victory that positively bridges the gap between where you are and where you want to be.

What's Your Motivation? The Quest for a Deep-Seated *Why*

Your *why* is one of the most crucial tools that you can count on when you are having trouble keeping your commitment to the 4-Week, 15-Minute Plan. In the beginning, after you've set your goals, you felt fired up and motivated, but in my experience with clients, after about three weeks, everything tends to become harder, and it's tough to keep going.

So, let's have a look at how you can make your *why* work for you when you feel yourself veering off course.

I always have goals, but my *why* is what keeps me focused. I have a belief that I'll take after my grandmother and live well into my nineties. If I'm lucky enough for this to be the case, I want to make sure that I'm fit, healthy, happy, and independent for as long as I can be, just as she was. My gran is my inspiration. That for me, is my deep *why*.

So embarking on the quest for your *why* is not just beneficial. It's crucial for lasting transfor- mation. It's the bedrock upon which sustainable change is built and the powerful antidote to the cycle of self-sabotage.

BEYOND THE SURFACE:
THE HEART OF YOUR *WHY*

I always say finding your *why* is a process. It's not a quick thought. Spend some time really thinking deeper than just the easy "I want to lose weight" as your *why*. There's always a deeper reason you want to start this journey. Your *why* must go beyond superficial desires. It's not about vague aspirations like easing menopause symptoms or wanting to tone up. It's the poignant reasons beneath these wishes that truly drive change.

THE EMOTIONAL CORE:
CONNECTING WITH YOUR *WHY*

Your *why* is rooted in the emotional aspects of your life. Maybe you want to play with your grandchildren with plenty of energy and without aches and pains. Or you may worry that your menopause symptoms are causing issues at work. You're having trouble focusing because of brain fog, inopportune hot flashes make you miserable, and your confidence is at an all-time low. Perhaps your relationship is suffering because you have no desire for sex, or you feel self-conscious due to extra weight gain and now your partner is feeling rejected. You fear that there is no way back for you both unless you make some changes.

This is how to connect with your *why*. It's unique to you and has to really mean something more than something just surface level.

THE PERSONAL IMPACT:
YOUR *WHY* IN DAILY LIFE

Examine how your menopausal symptoms are shaping your life. Is it impacting your intimate relationships, your self-esteem, or your professional performance? Your *why* should reflect these deeper, more personal stakes. You may have more than one *why*, but there will always be a common denominator. Find it and keep that at the forefront of your mind.

A CONSTANT REMINDER:
KEEPING YOUR *WHY* VISIBLE

Once you've identified your true *why*, make it a visible part of your everyday life. Write it down, place it where it can't be ignored, like putting a sticky note on your mirror or closet door, and let it be the first thing you see each day. This will be a reminder throughout your day to keep you on track. Otherwise, it's easy to forget in your busy life. Even if you think you haven't read the message, just having it there acts as a subliminal message for you without you realizing.

THE INNER DRIVE:
YOUR *WHY* AS YOUR COMPASS

Always use your *why* as the thing that directs you to where you want to go. Let it serve as your compass and keep it firmly etched in your mind. On days when the path is difficult, when old habits beckon, your *why* will be the spark that reignites your commitment to yourself and steers you back on course.

YOU DESERVE GOOD THINGS:
EMBRACING YOUR *WHY*

We can so easily believe we don't deserve to be in a better place than where we are right now. Remember, your *why* is a reminder of your worth and the life you deserve to lead. It's the affirmation that feeling better isn't just a desire. It's something you deserve, a state of being that you are fully entitled to pursue.

It's a good idea to begin to get clear on your *why* now because you'll need this reason to motivate you as you begin Week 1 of the program. We'll talk about this more in the next chapter.

Embracing Balance: The 80/20 Rule for Sustainable Progress

Now that you have your *why* (or are working on it!), it's time to learn more about the 80/20 rule. It's not just a strategy. It's a commitment to balanced enjoyment and healthiness. It's about nourishing your life with choices that serve you well, while also allowing room for flexibility and joy.

For me, this has been a complete game-changer because when I'd deprive myself, I always felt like I was missing out. This happened if my family was enjoying a lovely meal while I was meticulously counting calories or drinking water when my girl-friends were having a glass of wine on a night out. Usually, my willpower waned and I'd say, "Oh, what the heck," and end up eating or drinking twice as much!

When I decided to enjoy these moments rather than feeling miserable, something amazing happened. I didn't overdo it, and I ended up making better choices and not feeling guilty. This is the mindset I want for you too. I always say, "We are too old to be miserable; life is for living and making memories." So, let's have a look how you can achieve this and still stay on track with your goals.

LIVING FULLY WITHOUT FEELING DEPRIVED: THE 80 PERCENT COMMITMENT

Eighty percent of the time, you'll want to focus on what enhances your health and happiness. This is your foundation, the bedrock of habits that contribute to your physical fitness and help manage menopause gracefully, for example:

- Taking a walk outside
- Doing a fifteen-minute workout
- Drinking your eight glasses of water each day
- Completing a ten-minute meditation
- Connecting with your girlfriends
- Writing daily in your journal
- Stretching your body
- Not snacking late into the evening
- Limiting your screen time before bed

LIFE IS UNPREDICTABLE: 20 PERCENT MATTERS

Think of the 20 percent as your wiggle room. Life happens, and you'll always be thrown curve balls. Succeeding is not about never having issues to deal with, but how you handle them. You'll have bad days, and you'll have stress in your life. There will always be birthdays, weddings, barbecues, vacations, and family engagements you'll have to navigate. On these occasions, focus on making happy memories rather than an underlying feeling of guilt if you eat, drink, or do something that you think is not part of the plan.

Life is unpredictable, and it's the 20 percent that accommodates the unexpected. This wiggle room gives you the freedom to live life without the rigid constraints that often lead to rebellion against your own goals.

CELEBRATING WITHOUT THE GUILT: GRACE IN THE 20 PERCENT

When you adopt an 80/20 mindset, you tell your-self that you are allowed to have the occasional treat. This curbs the desire to overindulge. Think about a child when you tell them that they are not allowed any candy. There's an inevitable tantrum. It's the same thing when you say *no* to yourself. You want that thing even more. It's human nature.

When you want to celebrate, for example, that's within this 20 percent. Savor that glass of wine or special meal or enjoy a slice of cake. Embracing these moments without guilt means making better choices overall, choosing enjoyment without excess.

THE 80/20 RULE: YOUR SAFETY NET

If you tell yourself that you are never going to overindulge occasionally, then you are kidding yourself. We all do this, me included. The key is not to never overindulge, but to pick yourself back up the next day and get back to doing what serves your healthy life.

Should you indulge more than planned, the 80/20 rule is your safety net. It's the understanding that perfection is not the goal, resilience is. Rather than succumbing to guilt, you simply return to your supportive habits the next day.

CONSISTENCY OVER PERFECTION: THE LONG GAME

We all know that consistency is key, but it's human nature to look for magic solutions. I know I did this for years. It was only when I made the decision to consistently choose healthy actions 80 percent of the time that results came.

When you make small goals or promises and take consistent action, you'll see changes not just in your mindset but also in your body and menopause symptoms. This has worked for me and so many of the women that I've worked with. The 80/20 split allows us to stay consistent and feel great about the choices we make because we have wiggle room for the occasional indulgence.

This approach emphasizes consistency over perfection. By sticking to your beneficial routines most of the time, you create a buffer for the occasional diversion, ensuring that these moments won't derail your overall journey.

CREATING JOYFUL MEMORIES: THE TRUE SPIRIT OF THE 20 PERCENT

Who wants to be on their deathbed knowing that they have missed out on making memories with family and friends because they were too scared that they would make a mistake and overindulge? No one! Changing your mindset allows you to not feel guilty, and you'll make better choices with your 20 percent. I guarantee it.

Ultimately, this rule is about creating memories and experiences that enrich your life. It's an invitation to live fully, with the wisdom that deprivation leads to discontent while mindful indulgence brings happiness.

The Art of Addition: Cultivating Abundance in Menopause

Embracing a mindset of abundance during menopause is also important and can truly be transformational. It's a positive mindset that focuses on what you want to add to your life, not what you must subtract. When you add healthy habits, it naturally displaces less beneficial ones, leading to a more fulfilling and sustainable lifestyle.

BECOMING MORE MINDFUL: ADDING PRACTICES TO NOURISH BODY, MIND, AND SPIRIT

Infusing your routine with positive practices, be it a morning walk, a short burst of exercise, or a nutritious meal, doesn't just improve physical health, it also nourishes the soul. By adding these elements, you gradually create less room for the habits that don't serve you well.

Adding good habits like drinking water not only quenches thirst but can also curb cravings for less healthy options. Similarly, integrating mindfulness practices like meditation (you'll find practices and resources in chapter 6) can quench stress and add a layer of calm and control to your day, helping to manage stress, a common trigger for unhelpful eating habits.

THE JOURNEY OF JOYFUL MOVEMENT: EXERCISE AS A GIFT

It's important to also change the way you think about exercise. How many times have you thought, "I really should exercise"? It's time to revamp that way of thinking.

You get to exercise! There are so many people in this world who don't have the luxury of moving their body. They would love to get up and do a workout but physically can't. If you are one of the lucky ones, it's time to change the narrative.

View exercise as a gift, not a chore. Making a habit of incorporating movement into your life should be about celebrating what your body can do, not punishing it for what you've eaten. By shifting to this perspective, exercise becomes a joyful addition rather than a punitive measure.

NOURISHMENT OVER DEPRIVATION: SAVORING THE GOOD

This philosophy also extends to food. We are lucky enough to have a whole array of nutritious foods that will fuel our body at our fingertips. Instead of grumbling at the thought of a plate of nutritious food because it isn't the fast food you always chose to think of as a treat, look at the nutritious plate of food knowing that is going to make you feel energized and full of life.

When you focus on the flavorful, nutrient-dense foods you can add to your plate, you naturally start to crowd out the less nutritious options. There's no room for feeling deprived when your meal is both satisfying and health-promoting.

BUILDING A SUSTAINABLE LIFESTYLE: ENJOYMENT AS THE FOUNDATION

How many times have you searched for quick fixes or magic solutions for your weight goals or menopause

Client Success Story

Cara's 4-Week, 15-Minute fitness approach was perfect for me. It provided support for my mental as well as physical well-being at a time when I needed it most. —KATH

symptoms? If you're like me, you've lost count. Over the years, I realized that there are no quick fixes or magic solutions. It all comes down to plain-old consistency with your workouts and nutrition. It's also about learning to love the process, finding things you enjoy along the way, and developing good habits that naturally eliminate bad habits.

Quick fixes are fleeting, but a new lifestyle built on positive habits is something you can count on. Remember, to create lasting change, smaller, consistent steps are key. Setting grandiose goals can lead to feeling overwhelmed, but attainable, daily actions build the steady momentum that forges lasting change. By shifting focus from deprivation to addition, from scarcity to abundance, we foster a mindset that celebrates each positive choice as a stepping stone to heightened wellness.

Embrace the 80/20 rule and allow yourself the flexibility to live life's unplanned moments without guilt. It's in this balance that happiness and health coexist harmoniously. Let go of the all or nothing approach and instead, cultivate a lifestyle that's robust enough to withstand life's ebbs and flows.

As you move through menopause, changing your mindset will help you feel more motivated and focused. Remember, you're not losing anything. You're adding practices that improve health and wellness and will make your life richer and more fulfilling.

Ultimately, switching to an abundance mindset will allow you to confidently move toward your goals and create the life you deserve. Menopause is an evolutionary time, and how we handle it is greatly affected by our perspective. Often, this phase of life is painted with a brush of loss and limitation, but viewed the right way, it can be a blank canvas for new growth and enrichment.

Action Steps

1 **Buy yourself a journal.**

2 **Write down your mid-term** and long-term goals.

3 **Visualize yourself** achieving your goals in each area of your life.

4 **Don't be afraid of wanting** more for yourself, so dream big.

5 **Learn to say *no*** to the things in your life that do not fill you up. Set your boundaries and put yourself at the top of your list of priorities.

6 **Begin thinking about your *why*.** This is your compass, the deep-seated purpose that will keep you on track.

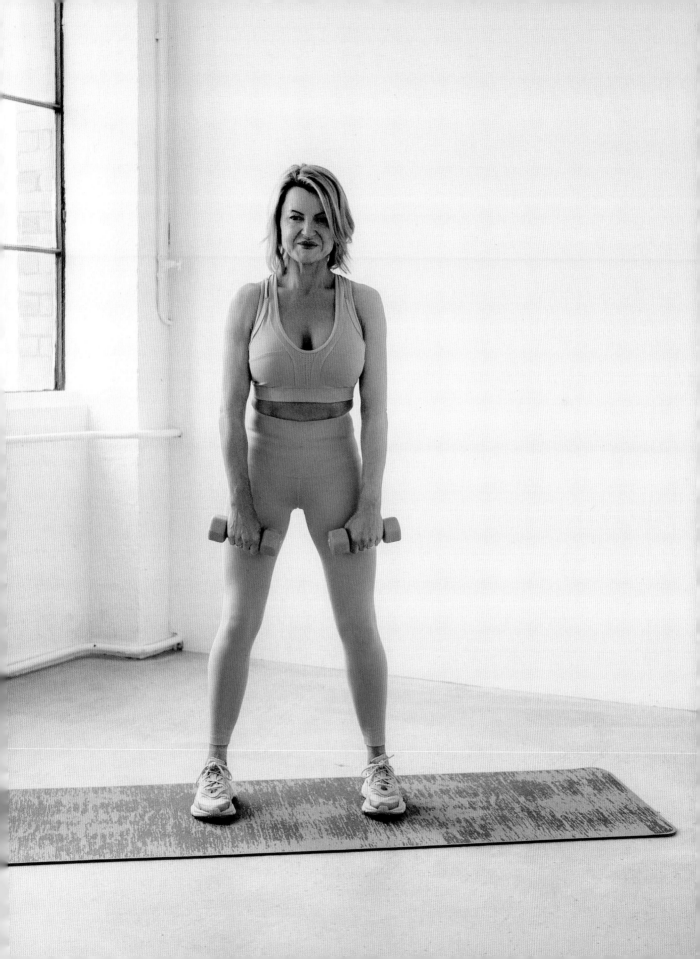

PART
TWO

Strength and Serenity:
The 4-Week, 15-Minute Transformational Plan for Menopausal Wellness

8

Let's Get Moving and More

Welcome to your 4-Week, 15-Minute Plan, specifically crafted for menopausal women. This journey is designed to empower you through an evolving period, focusing on holistic wellness and strength. Each week, we'll explore a variety of exercises, from strength training with weights to mindful meditation and targeted workouts like Abs and Body Sculpt.

My aim is to make each week simple and manageable and to build in intensity as you go. I'll push you to work hard, but at the same time, you'll have my understanding of the challenges menopause can give.

Recognizing the unique challenges of menopause, this plan is tailored to not only address physical health but also to nurture mental and emotional serenity. The aim is to provide you with the tools and routines that will help you manage menopause symptoms effectively, improve your overall health, and instill a sense of empowerment and vitality. Let's embark on this journey together, embracing each step toward a healthier, stronger, and more balanced you.

The 4-Week, 15-Minute Plan: Weeks 1–4

You'll see that each week increases with intensity. You may feel that in Week 1 there is not enough with regards to working out. This has been deliberate. How many times have you started a regime all guns blazing and fallen and given up in Week 3?

In my experience, this is the time that most people will give up. Motivation disappears and life gets in the way. We need to build habits and create a new mindset, and that comes with time and practice.

Remember those small goals?

They start here in Week 1. Start small and you will succeed! First, take a look at an overview of the 4-Week, 15-Minute Plan schedule. Here's what to expect week by week:

The 4-Week, 15-Minute Plan Schedule

Week 1

Day 1 Food journal and find your *why*!

Day 2 Walk outside

Day 3 Stretch—Body Flow

Day 4 Rest

Day 5 Workout—Weights 1

Day 6 Meditation—visualize your best self

Day 7 Rest

Week 2

Day 1 Workout—Body Mix 1

Day 2 Stretch—Body Flow

Day 3 Workout—Pelvic Floor and Abs

Day 4 Walk outside

Day 5 Workout—Weights 2

Day 6 Meditation—Breathwork

Day 7 Rest

Week 3

Day 1 Workout—Body Sculpt 1

Day 2 Walk outside

Day 3 Workout— Weights 3

Day 4 Stretch—Body Flow

Day 5 Workout—Abs 1

Day 6 Meditation—visualize your best self

Day 7 Rest

Week 4

Day 1 Workout—Weights 4

Day 2 Walk outside

Day 3 Workout—Abs 2

Day 4 Workout—Body Sculpt 2

Day 5 Workout—Body Mix 2

Day 6 Stretch—Body Flow

Day 7 Meditation—Breathwork

Week 1

Welcome to Week 1 of the 4-Week, 15-Minute Plan! Think of this as your journey to wellness. This week is all about building the groundwork for the transformative weeks ahead. We'll start by tuning into our bodies and minds through a food journal and identifying our deep *why*, which means understanding the true reasons behind our commitment to health.

You'll also learn more about important aspects of the plan, such as walking, workouts, meditation, and rest. Please trust the process starting with Week 1. You may feel you are not doing enough, but this is the foundation for the rest of your path to health and wellness.

Each Day Brings a New Focus

DAY 1. FOOD JOURNAL AND FIND YOUR *WHY*!

Begin by tracking what you eat and exploring the motivations that drive you. This introspective exercise isn't just about what's on your plate. It's about connecting with your health goals on a deeper level.

You may be ready and raring to go with a workout, but I want you to take one step at a time. Nutrition will be the difference between "okay" results and "amazing" results on this four-week journey. So please don't skip this part.

On day 1 of your journey, the cornerstone of our self-discovery is the seven-day food diary. This isn't merely a log of meals and beverages, it's a reflective journal that captures the intimate details of your daily well-being. As you document everything you consume and the times of your meals, also note your energy levels, your mood swings, any feelings of bloating, and even your anxiety levels. Record how you awaken each morning, the quality of your sleep, and every fluctuation in your status throughout the day. This is all super important. Awareness is key to knowing the changes you may need to make now and in the future.

The power of this diary lies in the patterns you'll uncover, linking the foods you eat to the emotions you experience and the energy you have. This clarity is pivotal as it guides you to make more informed choices that directly impact your menopause symptoms and overall health. You'll also find recipes in this book that will hopefully inspire you to create fabulous nutrition to feed your mind, body, and soul.

At the same time, dive into uncovering your *why*. This profound question isn't satisfied with superficial answers. It demands depth, seeking the core reason that will anchor you firmly to your path, even when distractions arise. It's time to dig deep and find what really makes you *want* to make changes and stick with this new way of life. This is all about mindset and understanding the deep reasons why we'll succeed, rather than throwing the towel in at the first hurdle.

Your *why* is your lighthouse in the fog. It's your steadfast companion when the journey gets tough. It's not just about "feeling better." It's about

Seven-Day Food Diary Chart

	WHEN YOU ATE	WHAT YOU ATE	HOW YOU FELT
Monday			
Tuesday			
Wednesday			
Thursday			
Friday			
Saturday			
Sunday			

What is your why?

ANSWER: _____

_____

_____

unearthing the compelling reason that resonates so deeply within you that it stops you in your tracks and steers you back on course whenever you stray. Once you're clear on your *why*, together we'll carve out a path to a healthier, more vibrant you.

If you need more help defining your *why*, review the sections in chapter 7.

DAY 2. WALK OUTSIDE

Adopt a simple, yet profound practice into your routine. Embrace the fresh air with a gentle walk outdoors. This is not just exercise. It's a way to celebrate your body's ability to move and breathe in the beauty of your surroundings. Even just a short walk will move you forward in the right direction, toward success.

Walking is far more than just physical exercise. It's an integral component of your wellness journey that engages both body and mind. As you step outdoors, you immerse yourself in the elements, which is rejuvenating on multiple levels. Even just ten minutes of walking in the natural light can significantly boost your vitamin D levels, essential not only for bone health but also for mood regulation and immune system support. The exposure to sunlight and fresh air helps to reset your internal clock, enhancing your sleep quality and circadian rhythms.

Walking is also a meditative act. With each step, you have the chance to clear mental clutter, reduce stress, and cultivate a mindset of mindfulness. The act of moving forward physically can be symbolic of progress in other areas of life, reinforcing a sense of direction and purpose. This time spent walking is an opportunity for gratitude, reflection, and connection to the environment around you. It's a grounding exercise that reminds you of the world's expansive beauty and your place within it.

Incorporating this simple act into your day can have profound effects on both your mental and physical state, making it a non-negotiable part of your health regimen. So, lace up your sneakers and step out. Your path to wellness is waiting right outside your door.

DAY 3. STRETCH-AND-FLOW

Gentle stretching encourages flexibility and helps to release tension throughout your body.

This practice goes beyond maintaining flexibility. It's about cultivating a serene mind-body connection. Mindful stretching helps manage cortisol levels, the stress hormone that, when elevated, can exacerbate menopause symptoms. By focusing on your breath and moving intentionally, you're not just enhancing your body's elasticity, you're also teaching yourself the art of controlled breathing, which can be a powerful tool for calming the mind and reducing stress.

Each stretch is an opportunity to listen to your body, to give space to areas of tightness and nurture flexibility. Keeping the body supple also helps to prevent injuries and improves posture and balance. For menopausal women, this gentle form of exercise is especially beneficial, providing a moment of tranquility in the day and supporting the body's natural processes in a time of change.

Embrace each movement, breathe deeply, and let the flow of the stretch be a guide to inner peace and lowered stress levels. See Body Flow on page 92 for this workout sequence.

DAY 4. REST

Rest is not merely a pause in your routine, but a vital component of your health and happiness, especially during the ever-changing period of menopause. It's on these days of rest that the magic of healing and strengthening happens. Your body uses this time to repair muscles, consolidate memory, and replenish energy stores, making rest as critical as any workout. So, think of rest like this, rather than thinking that you're being lazy. You need it sometimes.

Moreover, rest is a key ally in regulating hormones and managing menopause symptoms such as hot flashes, mood swings, and sleep disturbances. It's also when your mind gets a chance to decompress, process the day's experiences, and rejuvenate.

By embracing rest, you honor your body's natural rhythms and give yourself permission to recharge fully. It's an act of self-care that bolsters your resilience, both physically and emotionally, and supports sustained motivation and performance over time. When you do work out again, you'll be more energized and perform better, rather than being exhausted and having bad form, which can lead to injuries. Once you injure yourself, you'll be out of action for weeks, so the days when you need to rest are vital for your long-term health journey.

Rest days should be marked in your calendar with the same importance as your most intense workouts, for they are the silent supporters of your wellness journey. Remember, taking time to rest is not a sign of weakness but a wise strategy for long-term success and vitality. You're creating a lifestyle that you can sustain over a long period of time. Rest days will help you keep moving forward and are nothing to feel guilty about.

DAY 5. WORKOUT—WEIGHTS 1

Engage your muscles with a weight training session designed to build strength at a comfortable pace.

Incorporating weights into your workout routine is not just about building muscle. For menopausal women, it's a cornerstone of maintaining and enhancing overall health. Strength training is critical during menopause, a time when women are at increased risk for osteoporosis due to decreased bone density. Working out with weights stimulates bone growth, which helps in reducing the risk of fractures and osteoporosis.

Moreover, as we age, we naturally lose muscle mass. Regular weight-bearing exercises combat this decline, preserving and increasing muscle strength and endurance. This, in turn, aids in maintaining metabolism, which can help in weight management, a common concern during menopause.

Strength training also has a beneficial effect on body composition and can improve the quality of life by making daily tasks easier and thereby making you less prone to injury. A stronger body supports a more active and independent lifestyle. Strength isn't just physical, it translates into a sense of empowerment and confidence. A strong menopausal woman is indeed a powerful force, equipped to handle the changes her body is experiencing with strength and resilience.

If you're just starting out and need to build your confidence with using weights, I suggest starting light and focusing more on your technique. Two-pound (1-kg) dumbbells are a great place to start. Once you feel confident, then look at purchasing slightly heavier dumbbells and begin mixing and matching the weights in your workouts.

Challenge yourself, but make sure you are not compromising your form. Working out in front of a mirror will help you with this. This is exactly the way I managed to work up to using 7-, 9-, and 11-pound (3-, 4-, and 5-kg) weights.

See Weights 1 on page 92 for this workout sequence.

DAY 6. MEDITATION— VISUALIZE YOUR BEST SELF

Connect with your inner self through meditation (page 85). It's time to quiet the mind and find clarity and peace.

Including short, guided meditations in your workout routine is an invaluable and essential strategy during menopause. Meditation is a powerful tool for stress management, which is particularly beneficial during this time when the body's stress responses can be heightened due to hormonal fluctuations.

By engaging in meditation, you're helping to lower cortisol and adrenaline levels, the hormones associated with the body's "fight or flight" response. Elevated levels of these hormones can disrupt hormonal balance and contribute to various menopause symptoms, including weight gain, sleep disturbances, and mood swings.

Through meditation, you allow your body to enter a state of relaxation, which can mitigate these stress responses and promote a sense of calm and balance. This not only aids in managing the physiological aspects of menopause but also supports mental and emotional health, providing a space for you to connect with yourself and create inner peace. The guided aspect ensures that even those new to meditation can follow along and reap the benefits, making it an inclusive practice for all.

DAY 7. REST

Take another day to listen to your body's need for rest, reflect on the week's experiences, and prepare for the days ahead. A rest day can mean different things to different people. You may want to take a rest day and still take a walk or be a coach potato instead. It's your rest day so find what works best for you.

Remember, this is a journey of self-care and self-love. Every step you take is a step toward a healthier, happier you. Let's embrace this week with open hearts and a commitment to our well-being!

HOW TO . . .

Meditate and Visualize Your Best Self

This meditation is a tool to help you to visualize your best self and transform your dreams into reality.

- **Find a comfortable, quiet space** where you won't be disturbed. Sit in a relaxed position, either on a chair with your feet flat on the floor or cross-legged on a cushion. Place your hands on your knees or in your lap. Close your eyes.

- **Take a moment to acknowledge** your journey and the goals you would like to achieve.

- **Begin by taking three deep breaths.** Inhale slowly through your nose, feel your chest and belly rise, and exhale gently through your mouth, releasing any tension. Allow your breath to become natural and steady, anchoring you in the present moment.

- **Imagine a version of yourself** who has achieved your most significant goals. See yourself with clarity and detail: how you look, how you feel, and the expressions on your face. Notice the confidence, the joy, and the sense of fulfilment you have from this version of you.

- **Visualize the achievements** that have brought you to this point. See yourself overcoming challenges, making decisions that align with your highest good, and taking steps that lead you closer to your goals. Feel the sense of pride and accomplishment in your heart.

- **Focus on the emotions you feel** as your best self. Is it peace, happiness, confidence, or a sense of purpose? Allow these feelings to fill you, enveloping you in a warm, positive light.

- **Now, imagine a path** from where you are currently to where your best self is. See yourself walking this path with determination and grace, making progress and drawing closer to your goals with every step. Each breath you take brings you more alignment, clarity, and energy to pursue your dreams.

- **Silently repeat to yourself:** "I am on my path to becoming my best self. With each step, I move closer to achieving my goals. I trust the journey and embrace my power to create my reality."

- **Set a timer for ten minutes,** with a gentle alarm to bring awareness that the meditation is over. Go through each of the above points over those ten minutes. When you feel your thoughts start to wander, bring yourself back to your breath. Then, once refocused, come back to your best self-thoughts.

- **When you hear the meditation come to an end,** gently bring your awareness back to the present. Wiggle your fingers and toes, take a deep breath, and as you exhale, slowly open your eyes. Carry the image of your best self and the emotions of your achievements with you as you move forward in your day.

You'll find more information about how to meditate and additional resources in chapter 6.

Week 2

Welcome to Week 2 of the 4-Week, 15-Minute Plan! You have started your transformational journey to improved health and wellness. So, give yourself a well-deserved pat on the back for investing in yourself!

By this point, you're already probably feeling a change in your symptoms and energy. The good news is that wherever you are on your path, taking daily steps as part of my 4-Week, 15-Minute Plan *will* bring you wins and noticeable improvements as you continue. I've seen the results both for myself and my clients.

In Week 2, we'll ramp up the program even more as I give you new, but I promise, very doable practices and challenges that will reinforce your gains from Week 1. Both of these will help you make progress in terms of symptom management and in improved energy and vitality.

Here's What This Week Looks Like

You'll find detailed descriptions of what each workout includes on page 92.

Day 1. Workout—Body Mix 1
We'll diversify our routine with a mix of exercises that target different muscle groups, enhancing overall body strength and stamina.

Day 2. Stretch—Body Flow
Continue to nourish your flexibility with a sequence of stretches that promote a harmonious flow of energy throughout your body.

Day 3. Workout—Pelvic Floor and Abs
Focus on your core with exercises designed to strengthen the pelvic floor and abdominal muscles, crucial for your overall stamina.

Day 4. Walk Outside
Consistency is key! Enjoy another walk outdoors to clear your mind and appreciate your growing stamina and endurance.

Day 5. Workout—Weights 2
Build upon last week's session with a new set of weight exercises, pushing a bit further to build muscle and resilience.

Day 6. Meditation—Breathwork
As your body grows stronger, so does your mind. Continue your meditation practice to cultivate inner peace and mental clarity.

Day 7. Rest
Honor your body with rest, allowing it to recover, reset, recharge, and absorb the benefits of this week's activities. Reflect on your journey so far.

This week, you'll feel yourself getting stronger, not just physically but also in your resolve to continue your journey. Remember to listen to your body and move at a pace that feels right for you. Keep in mind that you're not just stepping up your efforts in terms of workouts and all the rest. You're elevating your entire constitution. So, let's keep moving forward together!

Week 3

Welcome to Week 3, a pivotal time in your 4-Week, 15-Minute Plan journey! This is when motivation can start to ebb, but it's also the moment to solidify the habits that will carry you toward a healthier life. This week is about digging deep, rekindling your inner fire, and reminding yourself of the *why* behind every effort you make.

Here's Your Plan for the Week

You'll find detailed descriptions of what each workout includes on page 92.

Day 1. Workout—Body Sculpt 1

Shape and tone your body with targeted exercises that focus on sculpting muscles, designed to empower you to feel strong and capable.

Day 2. Walk Outside

Continue your outdoor walks, using this time to reflect on your progress and reconnect with your goals.

Day 3. Workout—Weights 3

Introduce new challenges in your weight routine to continue building strength and endurance, pushing past your comfort zone.

Day 4. Stretch—Body Flow

Maintain your body's flexibility and fluidity with a series of stretches that also provide a mental break and stress relief.

Day 5. Workout—Abs 1

Strengthen your core with an abdominal-focused workout that is essential for back support and overall stability.

Day 6. Meditation—Visualize Your Best Self

As the intensity of your workouts increases, so does the need for mental balance. Use meditation (page 85) to ground yourself and maintain focus.

Day 7. Rest

Give your body the time it needs to recuperate and heal, ensuring you're ready for the days to come.

Week 3 will test your commitment, but every day you choose to continue, you're reinforcing a commitment to a healthier you. Keep pushing forward and remember that with each day, you're reducing menopause symptoms and improving your quality of life. Let's make this week count!

Week 4

Welcome to Week 4 of the 4-Week, 15-Minute Plan, which is the final stretch of our dedicated journey together! You've laid a strong foundation for a healthier lifestyle, and it's essential to recognize the power of the consistent effort you've put in. The habits you've developed are the bedrock for continuing your path to wellness, providing a blueprint for life beyond this plan.

Here's Your Focus for This Week

You'll find detailed descriptions of what each workout includes on page 92.

Day 1. Workout—Weights 4

Challenge your muscles with the most advanced weight training yet, designed to solidify the strength you've been building.

Day 2. Walk Outside

Take your walks as an opportunity to reflect on the progress you've made and to envision continuing this journey.

Day 3. Workout—Abs 2

Enhance your core strength with a second level of abdominal workouts, crucial for your body's central support system.

Day 4. Workout—Body Sculpt 2

Continue sculpting your physique with refined movements that aim to tone and define your body's contours.

Day 5. Workout—Body Mix 2

A varied routine keeps the body guessing and the mind engaged. Embrace this mix of exercises that target different areas.

Day 6. Stretch—Body Flow

Flexibility and mobility are just as important as strength. Use this session to elongate and soothe your muscles.

Day 7. Meditation—Breathwork

Conclude your week with your meditation practice to both balance the physical exertion and to center your thoughts on your achievements and goals.

Healthy Habits Mean Consistent Progress

Remember, consistency is key to your success. The habits you're creating now will carry forward, helping to make progress and to achieve and maintain the level of comfort you deserve. Remember, this isn't the end. It's the start of a lifestyle geared toward reducing menopause symptoms and promoting overall health. Next, we'll take a closer look at the specific workout routines in the 4-Week, 15-Minute Plan.

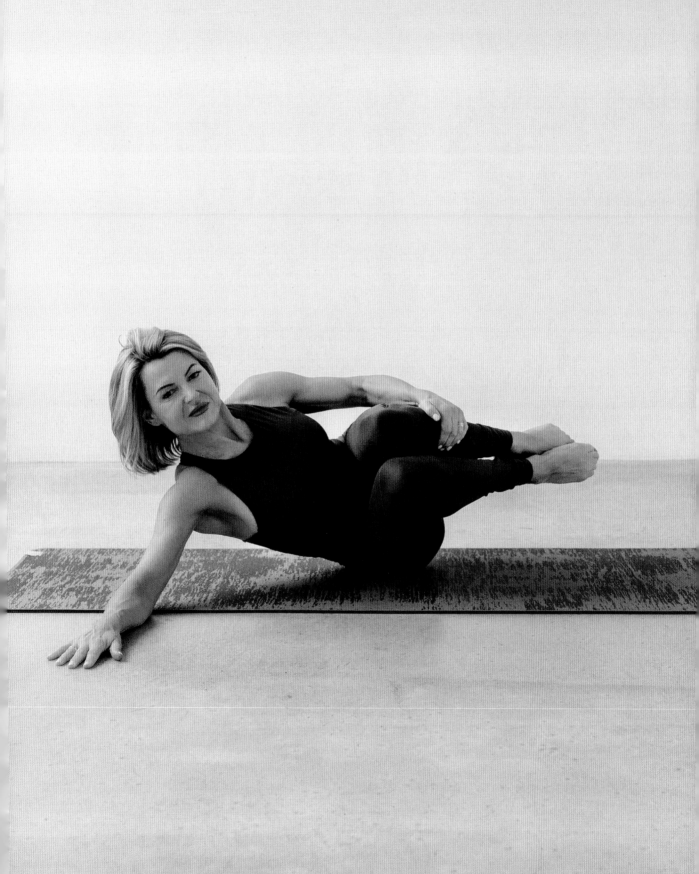

9

The 4-Week, 15-Minute Workouts

Body Mix Workouts

This was the workout that started off the Cara Fitness 15-Minute Method. I started this workout when I had no time to exercise, or I thought I had no time. Between dropping the children off to school, walking the dogs, and then getting ready for work, I had twenty minutes to spare.

So, I decided to give myself five minutes to get ready and to work out for fifteen minutes. I chose five exercises to target all areas of the body and repeated them three times. I made this my promise to myself each weekday, and that is how the method was born. Because I enjoyed the process, I could stay consistent and therefore got results. This is why I am so passionate about the 4-Week, 15-Minute Plan and my Body Mix Workouts.

The Body Mix Workouts are a key component of your exercise routine, thoughtfully designed to provide a comprehensive workout without overtaxing any single muscle group. This approach ensures that you can maintain proper form and technique throughout, which is crucial for preventing injury and maximizing the effectiveness of each movement.

By targeting five different areas of the body within a concise fifteen-minute session, these workouts are efficient and manageable, even for those with busy schedules or limited stamina. They strike the perfect balance between intensity and endurance, leaving you worked out but not worn out. The quick pace keeps the energy up and motivation high, allowing you to finish with a sense of accomplishment.

This type of workout is especially beneficial for menopausal women, as it boosts overall muscle engagement without leading to the kind of fatigue that can be discouraging and detrimental to form. It's an empowering way to fit in a full-body workout that enhances strength, coordination, and balance, all within a time frame that feels swift and satisfying.

Body Sculpt Workouts

I created Body Sculpt Workouts because I felt targeting two areas of the body in one workout would be powerful. By alternating from one area to the next, it allows the muscles to not fatigue too much, therefore helping to keep great technique.

The Body Sculpt Workouts are meticulously crafted to home in on two specific body areas, offering a targeted fifteen-minute session that maximizes strengthening and conditioning. This concentrated approach is highly effective for building lean muscle and enhancing muscular endurance in those specific areas, allowing for intense focus and measurable progress.

These sessions are brief but potent, designed to fit into your day without overtaking it. In just a quarter of an hour, you engage in a series of movements that not only challenge and fortify your muscles but also boost your metabolic rate, which is beneficial for overall health and weight management.

For menopausal women, Body Sculpt Workouts are particularly empowering. They not only help counteract the muscle loss and potential bone density reduction associated with menopause but also instill a sense of strength and achievement.

Completing these workouts leaves you feeling physically stronger and mentally invigorated, reinforcing a self-image of capability and resilience. It's a reminder that you have the power to shape not just your body, but your life's narrative, one rep at a time.

Abs Workouts

There is nothing like a great abdominal workout. Feeling the fire in your core is such a great feeling, knowing you are really working the epicenter of your body. That is why I have included some great Abs Workouts for you in this plan. They are simple, yet so effective. Mastering them will give you a great foundation for any core workouts you'll do in the future.

Abs Workouts are a cornerstone of fitness, especially for menopausal women, where the core's strength plays a pivotal role in overall health. A robust core is your body's powerhouse, providing stability and support for virtually every movement. These workouts are designed to build that central strength, ensuring your posture is upright and your movements are supported, which is essential for maintaining balance and reducing the risk of falls as you age.

Focusing on the core goes beyond the superficial muscles. It includes deep work on the pelvic floor, which is often neglected despite its importance. A strong pelvic floor is crucial for bladder control, sexual health, and lower back support. During menopause, hormonal changes can weaken these muscles, but targeted abdominal exercises can help to strengthen them, contributing to your body's overall function and vigor.

Incorporating Abs Workouts into your routine does more than improve physical health. It also brings a sense of control and empowerment. Knowing that you are taking proactive steps to maintain and enhance your body's core will give you confidence and peace of mind. It's an investment in your present and future health, ensuring you remain active, agile, and free from preventable core-related issues.

The 4-Week, 15-Minute Plan: Workout Sequences

For each week, you'll see workouts to focus on. Here, you'll find the sequence of exercises included in each one.

Each exercise is done for 50 seconds with a 10-second rest in between each. There are 5 exercises in each workout and the sequence is repeated 3 times to complete the 15-minute workout.

Body Flow consists of 10 stretches. Hold for 1 minute each, for a 10 minute stretching session.

The 4-Week, 15-Minute Plan Workout Schedule

WEIGHTS 1
1 Bicep Curl
2 Chest Press
3 Side Raise
4 Kickback
5 Shoulder Press

WEIGHTS 2
1 Front Crosses
2 Wide Scoop Up
3 Front Raise
4 Pec Dec
5 Triceps Extension

WEIGHTS 3
1 Front Raise
2 Bicep Curl
3 Upright Row
4 Kickback
5 Pec Dec

WEIGHTS 4
1 Chest Press
2 Front Crosses
3 Triceps Extension
4 Wide Scoop Up
5 Shoulder Press

BODY FLOW
1 Tabletop
2 Forward Fold
3 Downward Dog
4 Cat/Cow
5 Crocodile
6 Thread the Needle, right
7 Thread the Needle, left
8 Kneeling Lunge, right
9 Kneeling Lunge, left
10 Child's Pose

BODY MIX 1
1 Squat
2 Upright Row
3 Lunge
4 Lunge
5 Plank

BODY MIX 2
1 Kickback
2 Knee Repeater
3 Knee Repeater
4 Press Up
5 Ab Leg Crosses

PELVIC FLOOR AND ABS
1 Ab Breath
2 Pelvic Floor Squeeze
3 Crunch
4 Pelvic Floor Pulse
5 Pulsing Crunch

ABS 1
1 Crunch
2 Tabletop Toe Tap
3 Scissors
4 Side Crunch
5 Side Crunch

ABS 2
1 Crunch
2 Alternating Leg Extension
3 Scissors
4 Ab Leg Crosses
5 Plank

BODY SCULPT 1— TRICEPS AND ABS
1 Crunch
2 Seated Triceps Press
3 Alternating Leg Extension
4 Triceps Press Up
5 Mountain Climber

BODY SCULPT 2— LEGS AND SHOULDERS
1 Half Sit
2 Half Sit
3 Side Raise
4 Squat Pulse
5 Shoulder Press

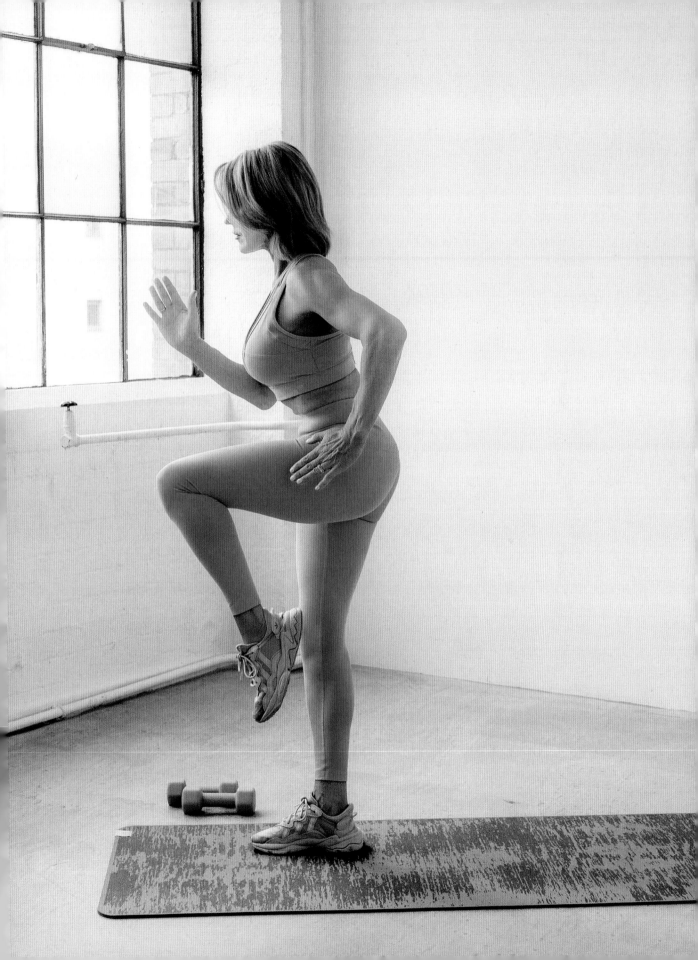

Bicep Curl

This is the perfect exercise to help with any lifting and carrying. It will make retail therapy even more satisfying as you'll be able to carry more bags.

Stand with your feet
hip-width apart.

Keep your elbows tucked
in to your body.

Breathe out as you
lift. Breathe in as
you lower.

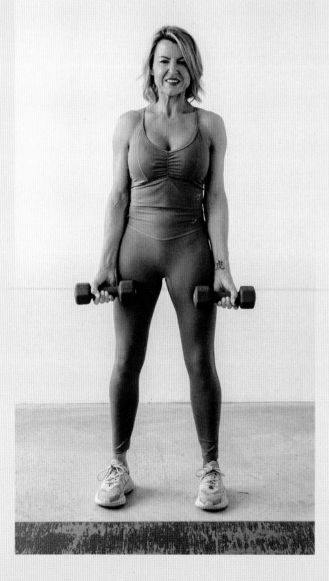
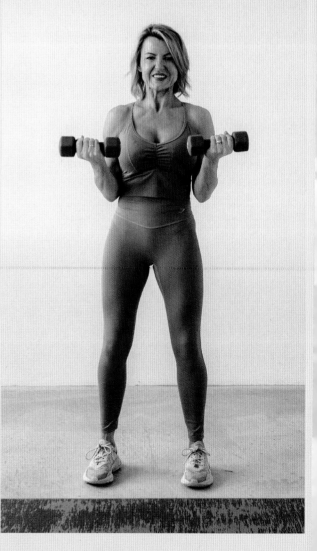

Chest Press

This challenging exercise will probably have you cursing me. However, you'll thank me for including this exercise when you are all perky and chest proud.

Stand with your feet hip-width apart.

Keep your fists shoulder height.

Brace your abdominals as you push the weights forward.

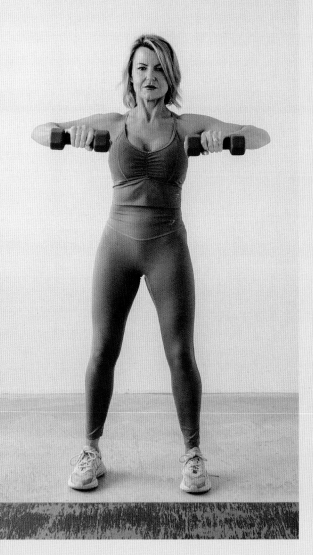

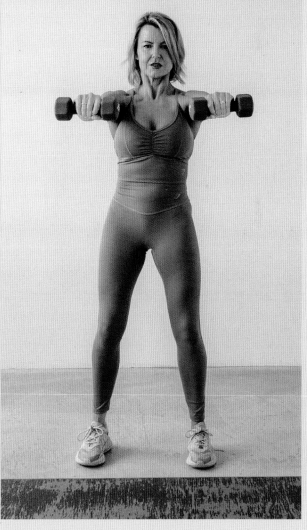

Side Raise

Have you ever wanted shapely shoulders? This simple exercise will give you just that—beautiful shoulders that you'll want to show off.

Stand with your feet hip-width apart.

Lean slightly forward, hinged at the hip.

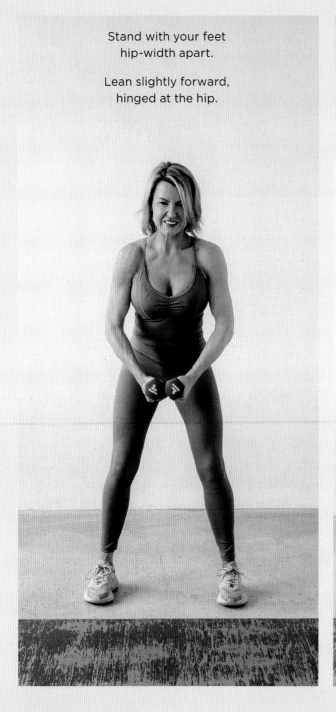

Keep your elbows slightly bent in a fixed position as you lift the weights.

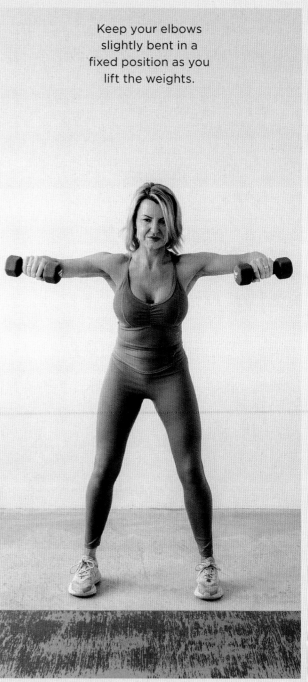

Squat Pulse

Are you ready to feel the burn in your thighs? If you can't feel it, you need to drop a little lower into the squat!

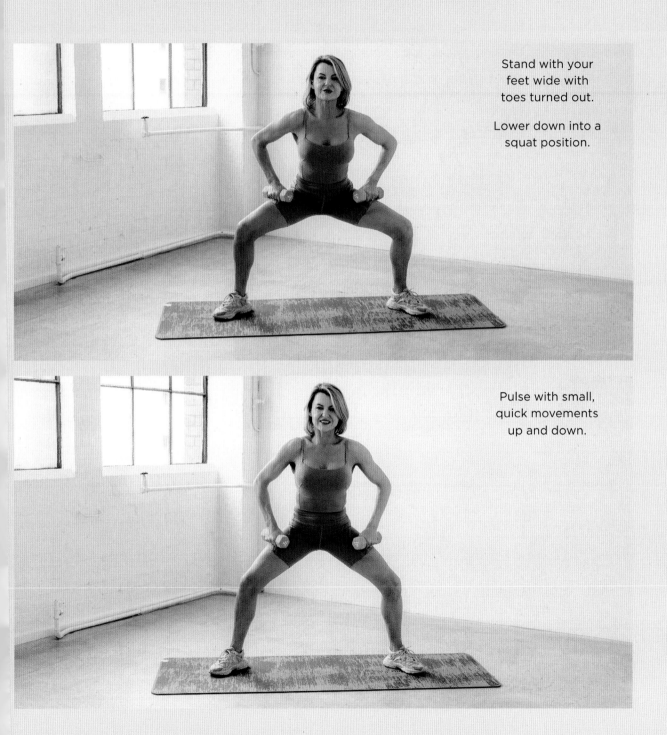

Stand with your feet wide with toes turned out.

Lower down into a squat position.

Pulse with small, quick movements up and down.

Kickback

I usually call exercises like this the "bingo wing" blaster, but thought
I better be a bit more serious. This exercise will tighten up the under-arm
and stop the wobble as you wave. Is that serious enough?

Stand with a split stance.

Lean slightly forward with
the elbows raised to
the back.

Extend at the elbows,
keeping the top of the
arm still as the arms
straighten.

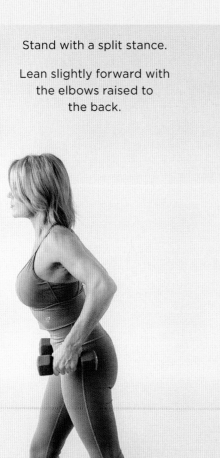

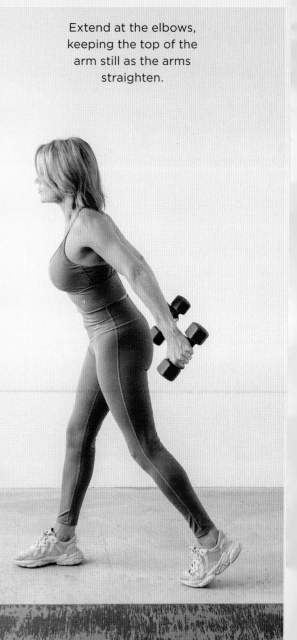

Shoulder Press

I love this exercise. Shoulder sculpting is one of my favorite things to do.
This exercise is simple but super challenging.

Stand with your feet
hip-width apart.

Look directly ahead as if
looking out to the horizon,
so your neck doesn't hurt.

Push the weight up and very
slightly forward so the weights
don't go behind your head.

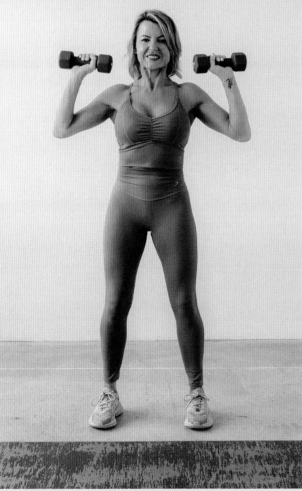

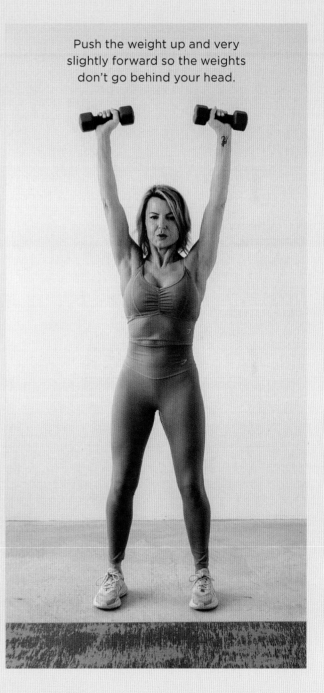

Front Crosses

Please be sure to make space when you cross the weights. Otherwise, you'll hit your hand with the crossing weight, and believe me, it really hurts!

Stand with your feet
hip-width apart.

Hinge slightly forward from
the hip. Start with the weights
at shoulder height.

Make plenty of space
when crossing the
weights, so as not to hit
your hands together.

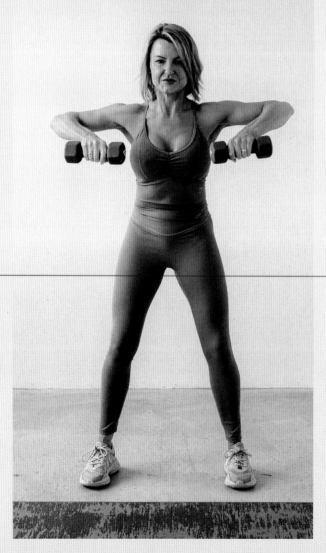
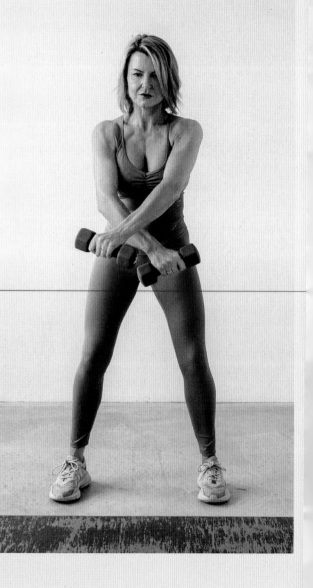

Wide Scoop Up

Imagine you are a wine bottle opener! Yes, you heard correctly. As your arms rise up, feel the energy in your body and shoulders compress down. Your arms are the arms of the bottle opener, and your body is the screw that goes into the cork. Doing this will make you feel strong.

Stand with your feet
hip-width apart.

Turn your palms upward
and scoop wide and up.

Breathe out and brace your
abdominals as you lift.

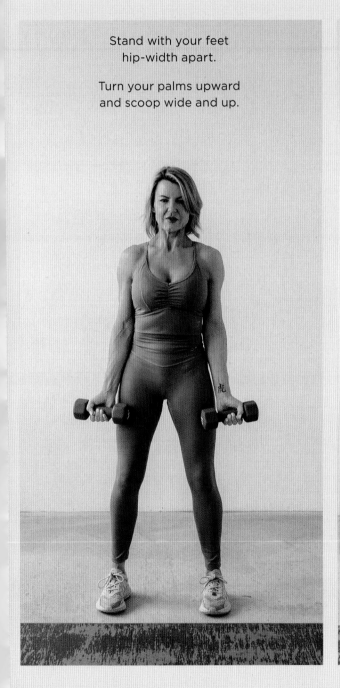
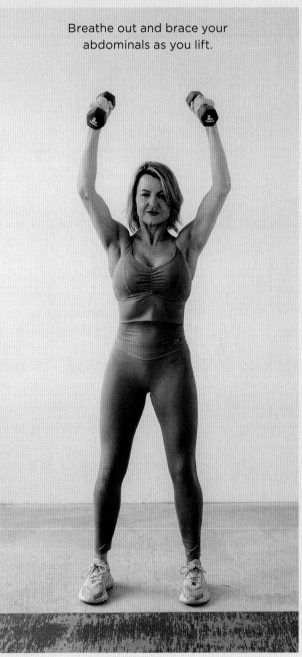

Front Raise

This great exercise will really make your abdominals work too.
Squeeze your abs as you lift the weights up. This will also stop your body
from swaying forward and backward, therefore protecting your back.

Stand with your feet
hip-width apart.

Turn your palms down and raise
your arms forward and up.

Breathe out and squeeze your
abdominals as you lift the weight.

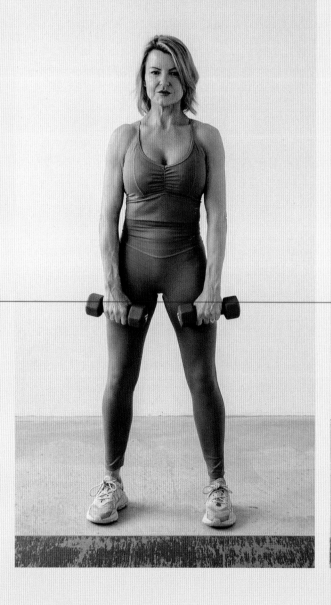

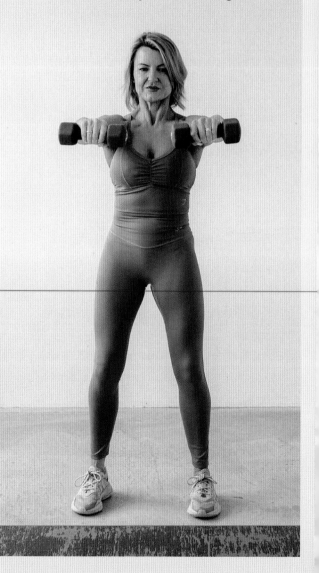

Pec Dec

This is the most challenging exercise in the weights section.
If at any time your neck hurts, please have a rest. Roll your shoulders
to loosen them before you get back to position.

Stand with your feet
hip-width apart.

Keep a 90-degree angle at the
elbow at shoulder height.

Try to bring the
forearms together while
you breathe out.

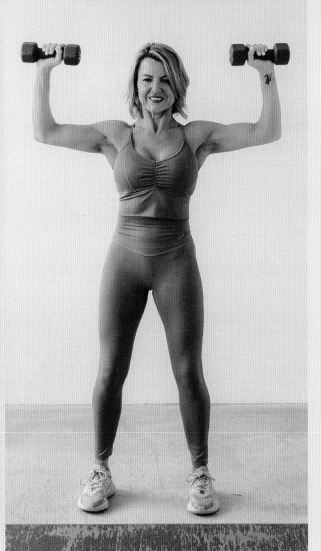
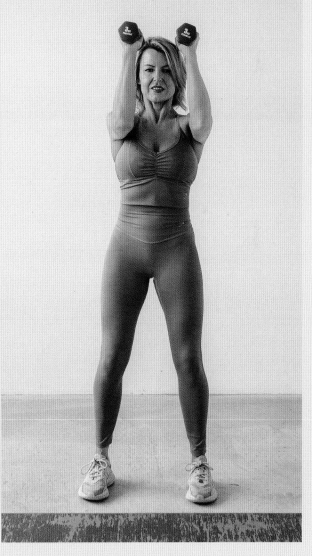

Triceps Extension

I love these "bingo wing" blaster exercises! This is no exception. I would highly recommend standing in front of a mirror to watch your form. My left arm is a little weaker than my right, and my left elbow tends to flare out, so I really have to watch myself. The key is to keep both elbows close to the head and really focus on your arm that may be the weakest.

Stand with a split stance.

Hold the weight in both hands above your head, keeping your elbows in line with your head.

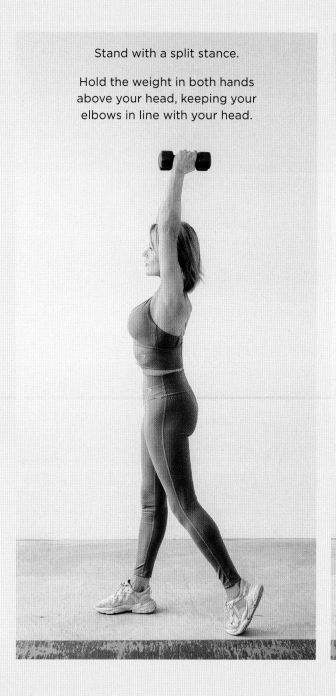

Lower the weight behind your head and keep the elbows as close to your head as possible.

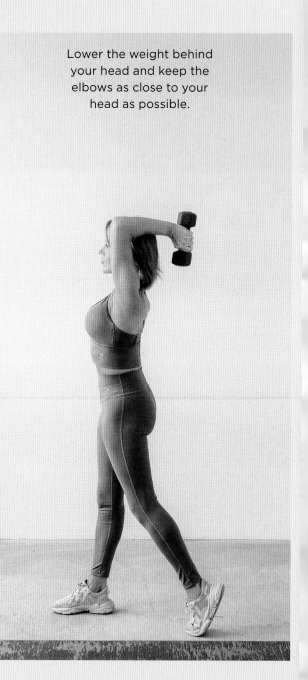

Upright Row

For this exercise, imagine you had a string tied to both elbows and you are a puppet. The puppet master pulls on the strings, and your elbows rise up. This way, you stop the weights coming up first, which puts pressure on your wrists. Let your elbows rise up and stay higher than your weights.

Stand with your feet hip-width apart.

Keep the weights close to the body as you pull the weights up.

Keep the elbows higher than the hands at all times.

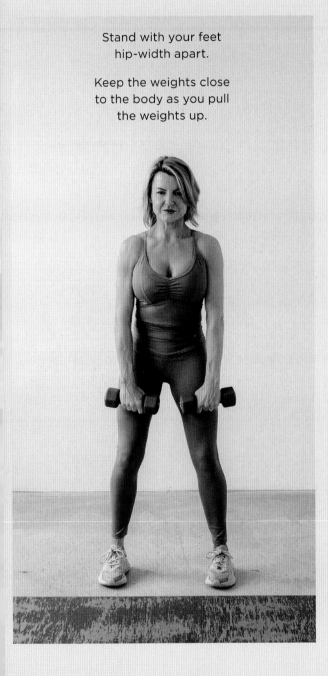
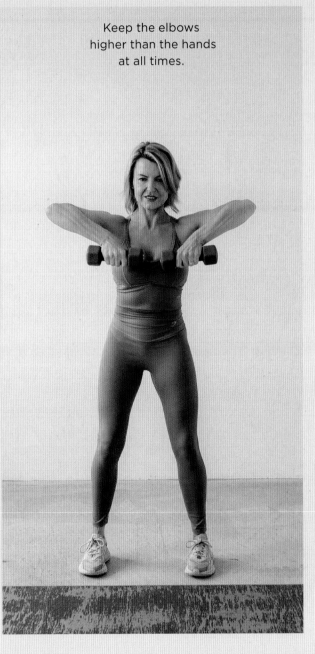

Tabletop

Not everyone can straighten their legs in this position and that's fine. Bend slightly at the knee if you need to. Try to have your weight over the whole of your foot so that you're not sitting back into your heels. This will maximize the stretch.

Hinge from the hip and pull the belly in.

Place the hands just above the knees for stability.

Breathe in through your nose and out through your mouth as you hold the stretch.

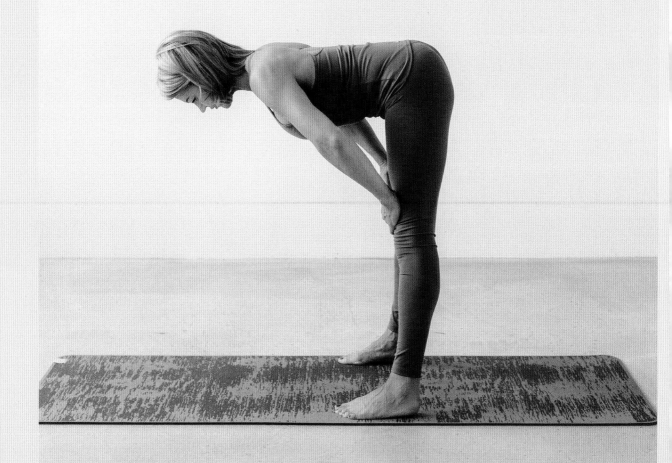

Forward Fold

With this exercise, you may need to bend your knees. Breathe into the stretch and allow your body to relax as much as possible. An important tip is to spread your toes out. The whole time you scrunch your toes up, tension will go through your foot, to the ankle and up the legs. Try to relax and breathe.

Hinge from the hip and reach
your hands to the floor.

Bend your knees to be able to
touch the floor.

Breathe in through your nose
and out through your mouth as
you hold the stretch.

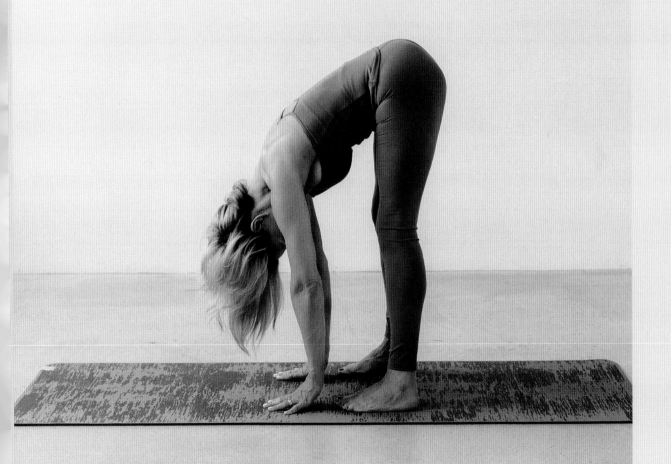

Downward Dog

This yoga pose helps increase flexibility in the hamstrings. Try to keep the heels to the floor if you can. Lift up through the hips, while you press down with your hands and heels. The two-way energy is a powerful force.

Place the palms of your hands to the floor so your body is in a *V* shape.

Try to keep the heels to the floor or as close as possible.

Breathe in through your nose and out through your mouth as you hold the stretch.

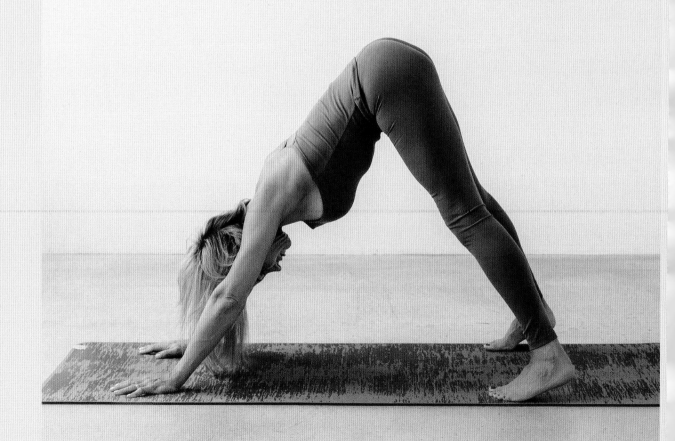

Cat/Cow

This is great for a stiff back. It's simple but effective and
helps release stress after a busy day.

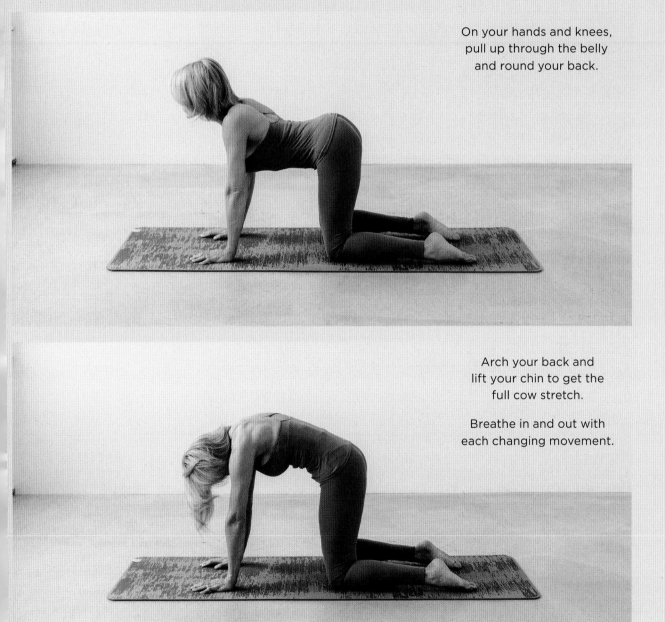

On your hands and knees,
pull up through the belly
and round your back.

Arch your back and
lift your chin to get the
full cow stretch.

Breathe in and out with
each changing movement.

Crocodile

I'll admit this is a tough yoga pose for me since I had spinal surgery. It's super important to do it though because it improves back flexibility and lengthens your hip flexors. I will keep doing this until I finally master it.

Lie with your belly to the floor and place your hands under your shoulders.

Push your chest away from the floor and look up to the ceiling.

Breathe into the stretch as you hold.

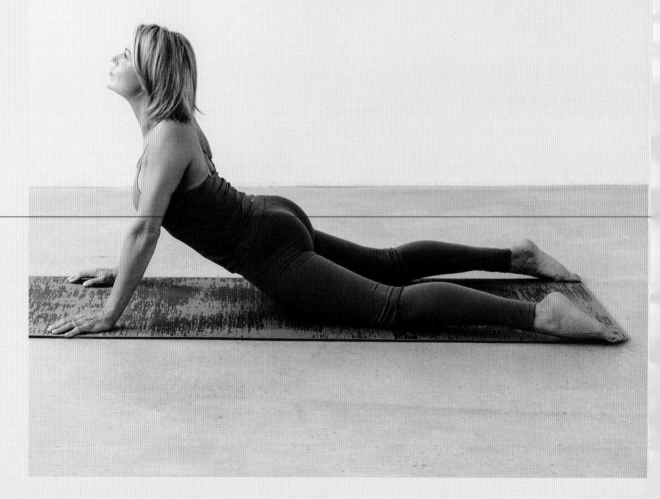

Thread the Needle

This is a great stretch for your shoulders and
increases rotation through the spine.

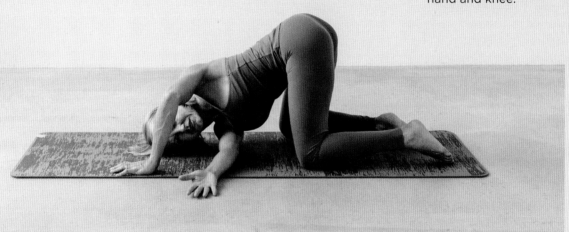

On your hands and knees,
thread one hand close to
the floor between your
hand and knee.

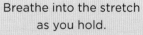

Try to keep your
shoulder to the floor as
you reach through.

Breathe into the stretch
as you hold.

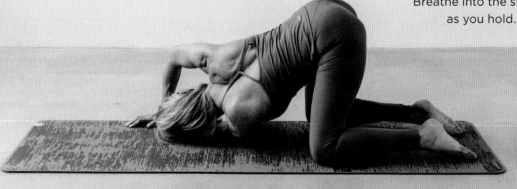

Kneeling Lunge

If you sit at a desk all day, you need this stretch. Tight hip flexors from sitting too long can cause all sorts of problems, especially back issues. Stretching the hip flexors will help alleviate this, so please make sure you don't skip this stretch.

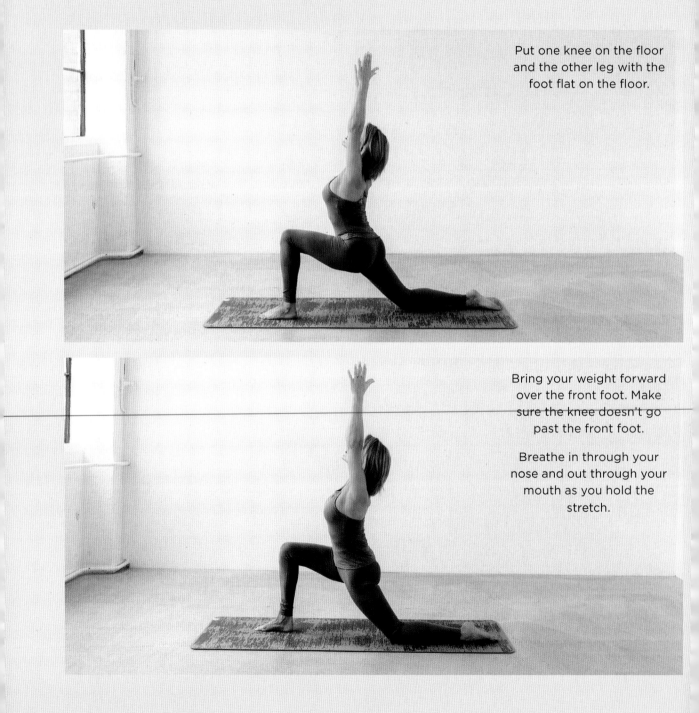

Put one knee on the floor and the other leg with the foot flat on the floor.

Bring your weight forward over the front foot. Make sure the knee doesn't go past the front foot.

Breathe in through your nose and out through your mouth as you hold the stretch.

Child's Pose

This is a calming and nurturing stretch. I like to press my hands into the floor
to feel a great stretch through the upper arm and armpit. You can also just
lightly touch the floor with your hands.

Start on your hands and knees.
Then, bring your feet together with the
knees wider than your hips.

Sit back toward your heels and reach
forward with your hands to the floor.

Take a deep breath and let go
into the stretch.

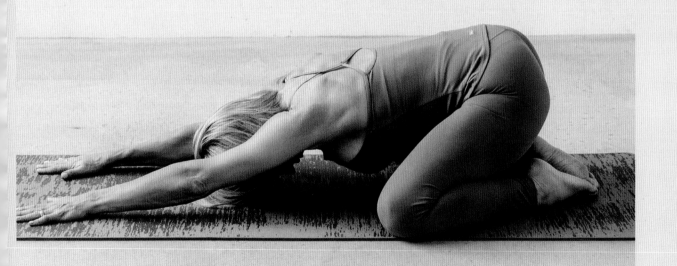

Squat

This versatile exercise can be done in many different ways: feet narrow, feet wide, toes turned out or feet straight. I love feet wide, toes turned out because it targets the inner thighs more. You may want to target your glutes more, so keep your feet straight. Feet narrow will really focus on the quads. Find your sweet spot.

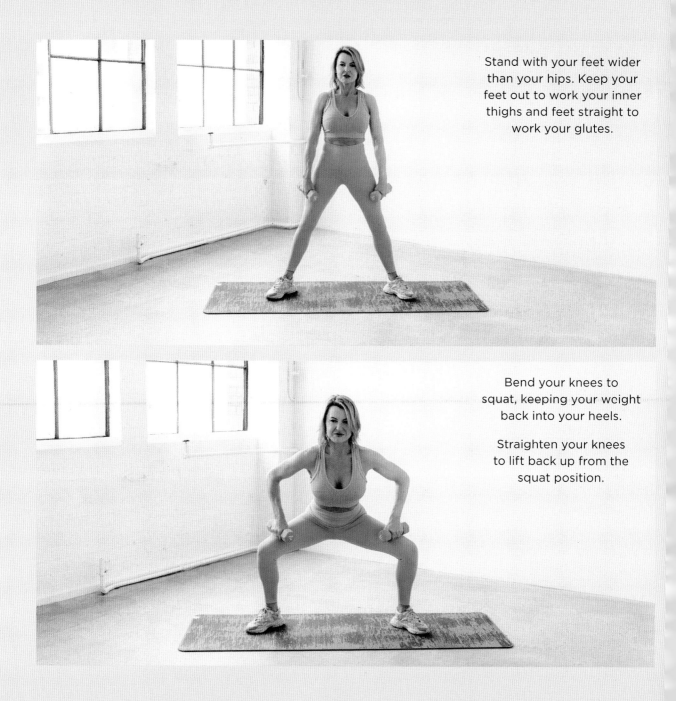

Stand with your feet wider than your hips. Keep your feet out to work your inner thighs and feet straight to work your glutes.

Bend your knees to squat, keeping your weight back into your heels.

Straighten your knees to lift back up from the squat position.

Lunge

I don't think I've ever heard anyone say they love doing lunges.
I know how great they are for the glutes and legs, so I love them,
but it doesn't mean I have to like them.

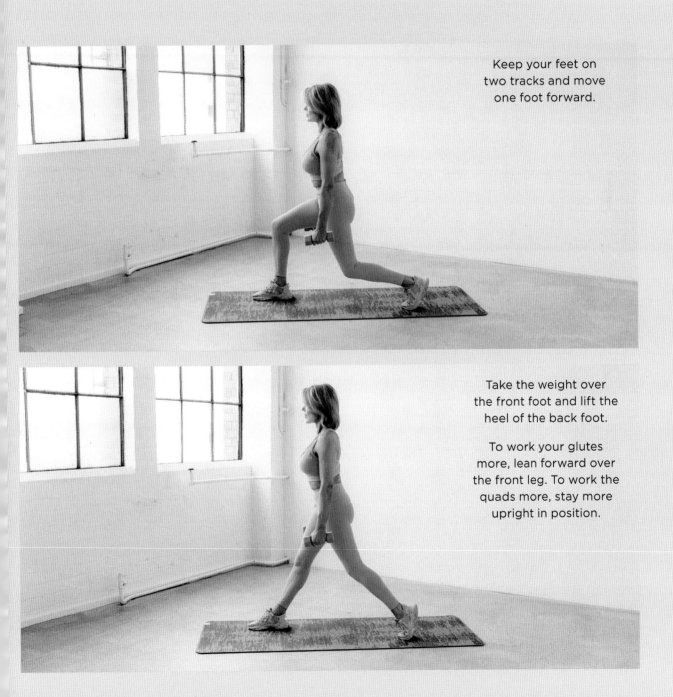

Keep your feet on
two tracks and move
one foot forward.

Take the weight over
the front foot and lift the
heel of the back foot.

To work your glutes
more, lean forward over
the front leg. To work the
quads more, stay more
upright in position.

Knee Repeater

This simple exercise is a silent assassin. You think when you start, "Oh, these are easy." However, when you get to 30 seconds, you'll feel differently. If not, sink deeper into the position, so you can really feel the burn.

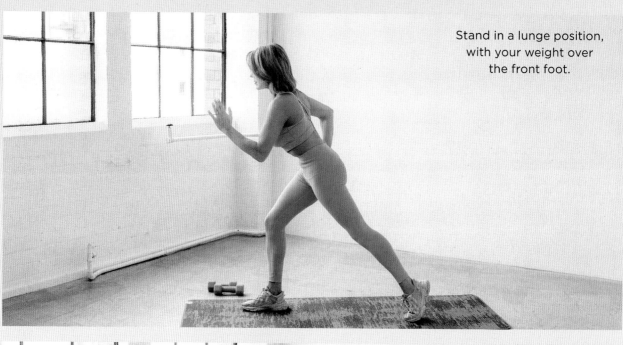

Stand in a lunge position, with your weight over the front foot.

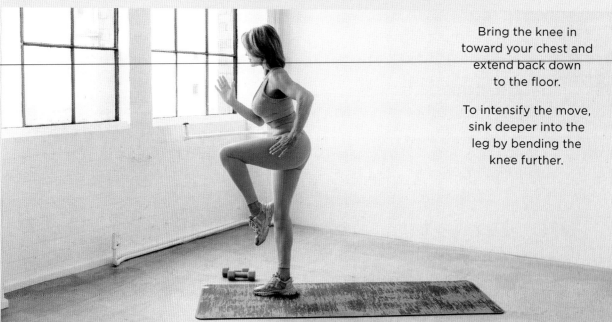

Bring the knee in toward your chest and extend back down to the floor.

To intensify the move, sink deeper into the leg by bending the knee further.

Press Up

It's best to do this one either from your knees or to place your hands
wide on the wall and press up from there instead.

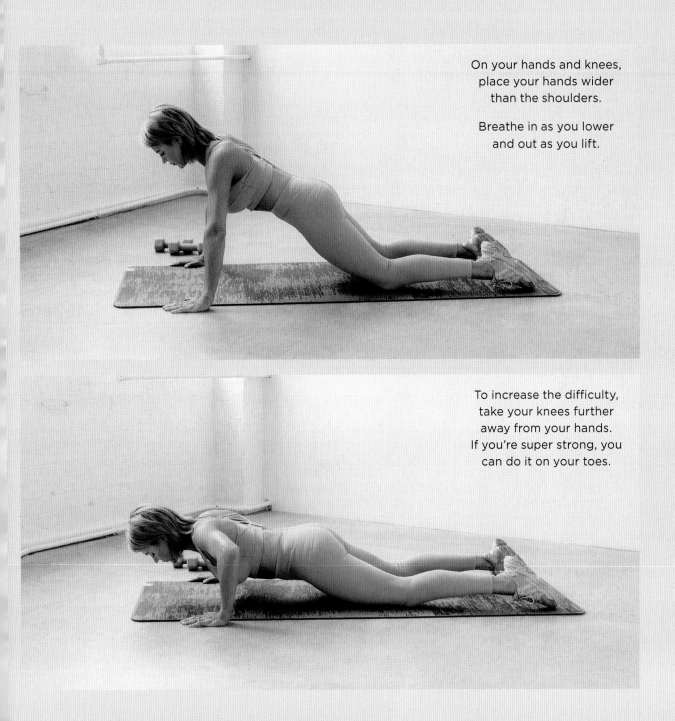

On your hands and knees,
place your hands wider
than the shoulders.

Breathe in as you lower
and out as you lift.

To increase the difficulty,
take your knees further
away from your hands.
If you're super strong, you
can do it on your toes.

Ab Breath

This is the base of all abdominal exercises. If your back or neck hurts while doing abdominal work, come back to this and breathe. You'll still be working your abs.

Lay on your back with your knees
bent and your feet flat to the floor.

Keep your spine in a neutral position.

Breathe in through your nose
and out through your mouth.
As you breathe out, pull your belly
button in toward your spine without
changing your neutral spine.

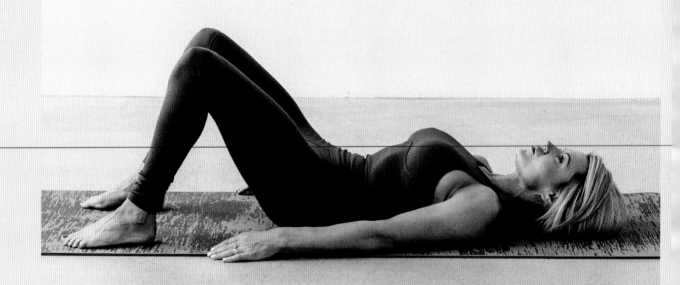

Pelvic Floor Squeeze

This is a tricky one but please bear with it. Really focus on where you are trying to work as it is vital to strengthen your pelvic floor so you can laugh and sneeze without worry!

Lay on your back with your knees bent and your feet flat to the floor.

Keep your spine in a neutral position.

As you breathe out, tighten and hold your pelvic floor muscles for 1 second and then release and repeat.

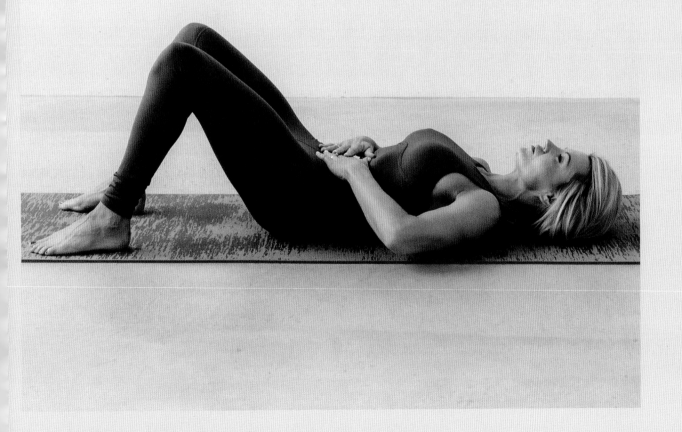

Crunch

This is probably one of the best known and least liked abdominal exercises. If your neck hurts when doing a crunch, it's important to breathe out as you lift the head and shoulders. Squeeze your abdominals at the same time. Don't worry about how high you get. Focus on how much you can squeeze your abdominals, particularly your lower abs.

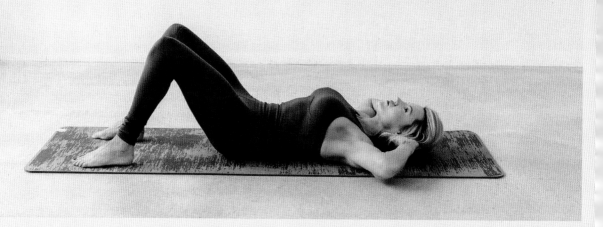

Lay on your back with your knees bent and feet flat, placing your hands lightly behind your head.

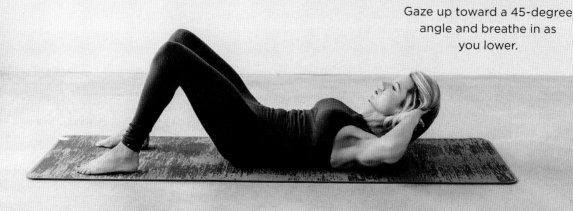

Take a deep breath in and as you breathe out, squeeze your abdominals and lift your head up.

Gaze up toward a 45-degree angle and breathe in as you lower.

Pelvic Floor Pulse

Little electric pulses are perfect for your pelvic floor pulse.
Focus, visualize, and squeeze like your life depends on it!

Lay on your back with your knees
bent and your feet flat to the floor.

Keep your spine in a neutral position.

Quickly tighten and release your
pelvic floor muscles.

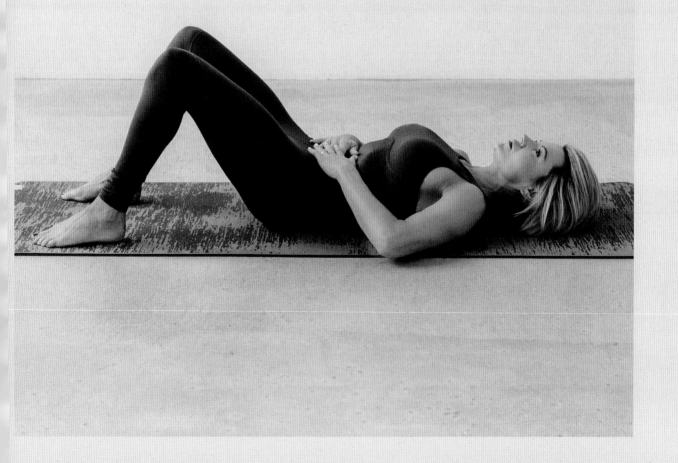

Pulsing Crunch

Imagine you have vacuum-packed your belly. Then, flatten as much as possible and squeeze and squeeze and you will really feel your abdominals working.

Lay on your back with your knees
bent and feet flat, placing your
hands lightly behind your head.

Take a deep breath in and
as you breathe out, squeeze your
abdominals, and lift your head up.

Pulse with small, quick
movements up and down.

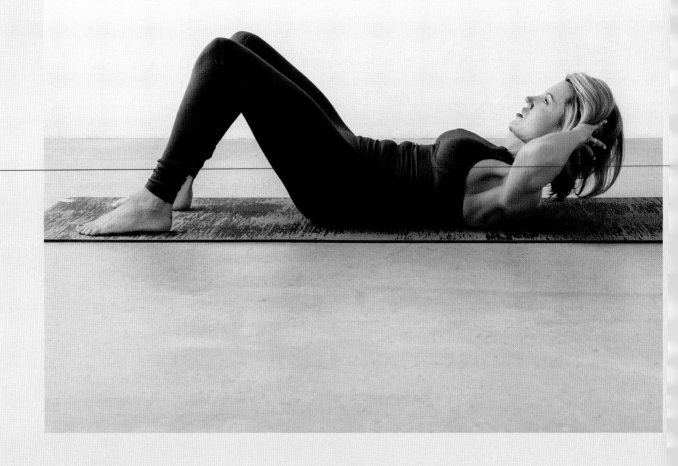

Ab Leg Crosses

This is a very challenging abdominal exercise. So, please always remember
you have choices. You can do it with your legs bent, legs straight, and your head
down or up. The further out and lower your legs are, the tougher it will be.
It's also more difficult with your head and shoulders off the floor. Choose what is
good for you by making sure it's only your abdominals that are working and
nothing else. If your neck hurts, take it down a level.

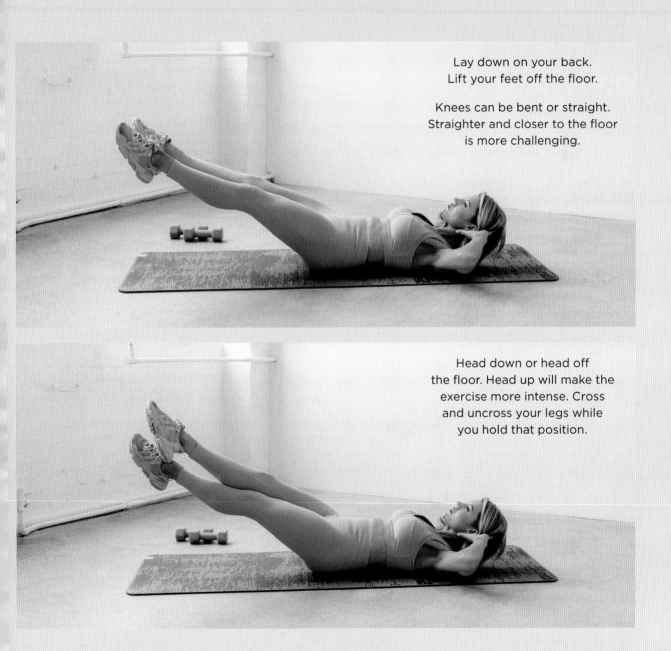

Lay down on your back.
Lift your feet off the floor.

Knees can be bent or straight.
Straighter and closer to the floor
is more challenging.

Head down or head off
the floor. Head up will make the
exercise more intense. Cross
and uncross your legs while
you hold that position.

Tabletop Toe Tap

This Pilates exercise looks easy but when done properly, can be so effective and very challenging. The key is to not let your knee come in toward your chest as you tap the alternating foot to the floor. Also, keep the angle at the knee the same. I like to imagine the legs are set in a plaster cast so the knees can't bend or straighten from the fixed position.

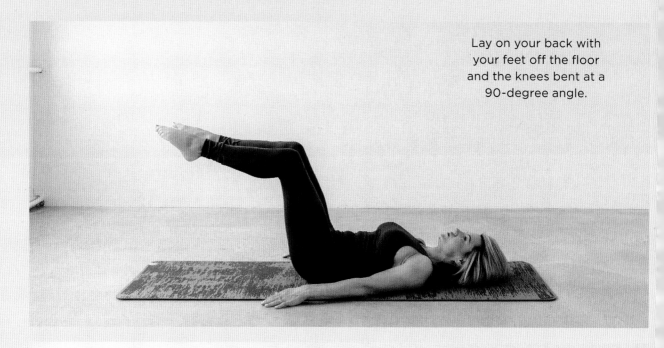

Lay on your back with your feet off the floor and the knees bent at a 90-degree angle.

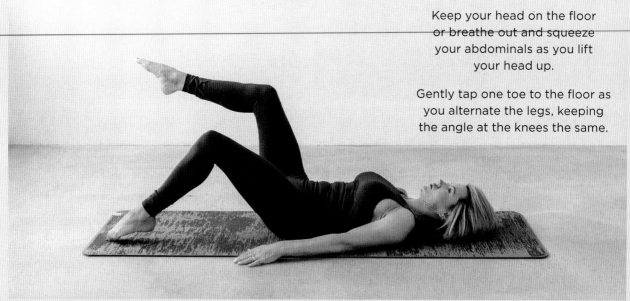

Keep your head on the floor or breathe out and squeeze your abdominals as you lift your head up.

Gently tap one toe to the floor as you alternate the legs, keeping the angle at the knees the same.

Scissors

This exercise is tough. You really need to focus on bracing your abdominals to stop your back from arching. If you feel it does arch, then please bring your legs to a more bent position or take a break.

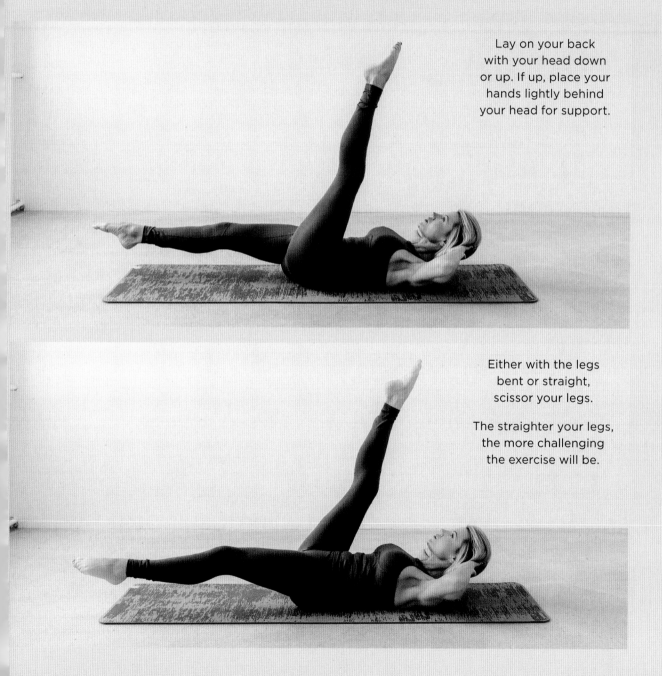

Lay on your back with your head down or up. If up, place your hands lightly behind your head for support.

Either with the legs bent or straight, scissor your legs.

The straighter your legs, the more challenging the exercise will be.

Side Crunch

I was not able to do both knees for the whole 50 seconds when I first started to do this exercise. To improve, I would do a little with a single knee and then a little with both knees. Eventually, I could manage both knees for 50 seconds. This is how to mix and match to increase the difficulty of an exercise.

Lay on your side with your hand stretched above your head.

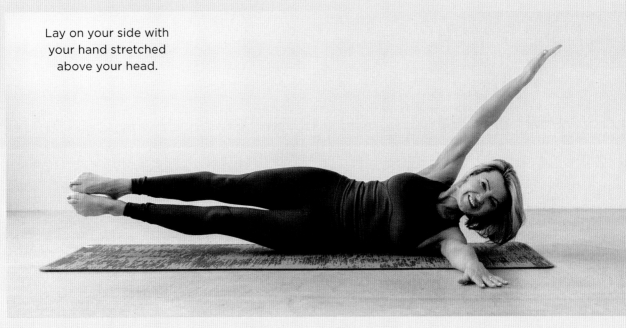

Bring either one knee in toward your chest or both knees in while lifting the body up toward your knee/knees.

Focus on your breath. Breathe in as you bring the movement in.

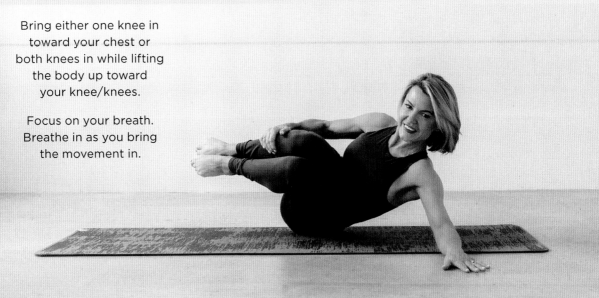

Alternating Leg Extension

This is easier for me than my lovely tall clients. Why? Because my legs are shorter. The longer your legs are, the tougher it will be.

Lie on your back with your head up or down.

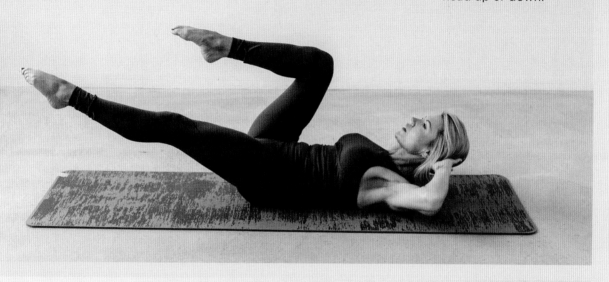

Bring one knee into the chest and extend the other, then alternate the leg positions.

Twisting the upper body to the knee will make the move more challenging.

Seated Triceps Press

You don't need any equipment for my favorite triceps exercise. You can also increase the intensity by pulsing down, slowing the speed, or just changing the rhythm of the exercise. It's very versatile and very effective.

Sit on your bottom with your hands slightly behind you and your fingers forward.

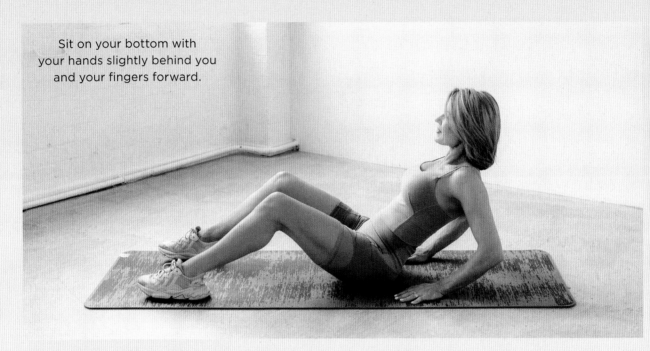

Bend the elbows as you breathe in and straighten the arms as you breathe out.

Keep the elbows narrow and in line when you lower to really work the backs of the arms.

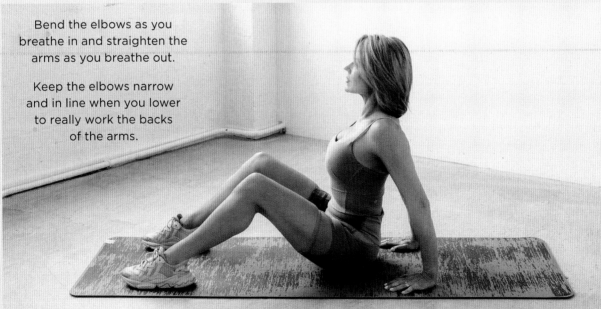

Triceps Press Up

This exercise is extremely challenging. Try imagining that you have a string tied to each shoulder and you have a hole in the center of each hand. Each string is threaded through each hand and then goes down through the floor to two little men below the floor. (Stay with me here!) The little men are pulling the string, making your shoulders go toward the back of your hands. This stops you from taking the weight back into your that legs, so you perform the exercise correctly. If you struggle, then don't go too far down until you get stronger.

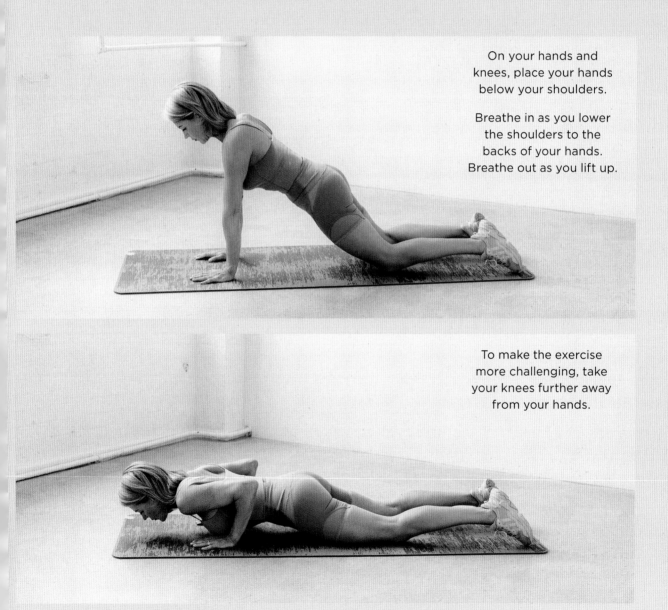

On your hands and knees, place your hands below your shoulders.

Breathe in as you lower the shoulders to the backs of your hands. Breathe out as you lift up.

To make the exercise more challenging, take your knees further away from your hands.

Mountain Climber

It's important to protect your wrists when doing this exercise. If you allow your shoulders to move forward past your fingertips, you'll put too much pressure on them. So, be mindful of your hands, shoulders, and wrists during this exercise.

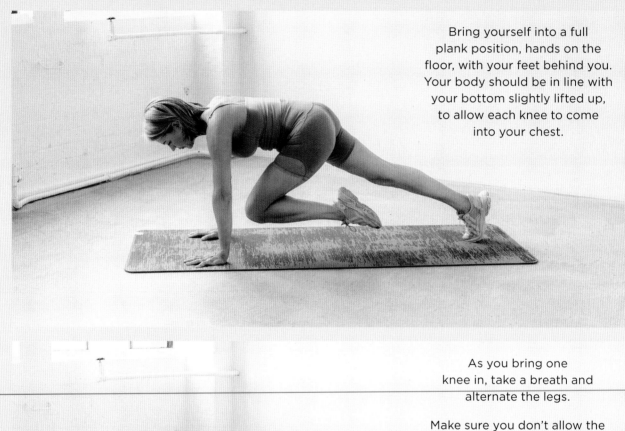

Bring yourself into a full plank position, hands on the floor, with your feet behind you. Your body should be in line with your bottom slightly lifted up, to allow each knee to come into your chest.

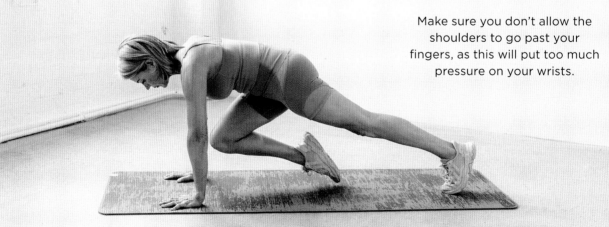

As you bring one knee in, take a breath and alternate the legs.

Make sure you don't allow the shoulders to go past your fingers, as this will put too much pressure on your wrists.

Half Sit

This exercise looks easy, but it's not. You'll see that it's the tiny pulsing movement that is the killer move. Your legs and backside will be on fire after this.

Stand with one foot slightly in front of the other.

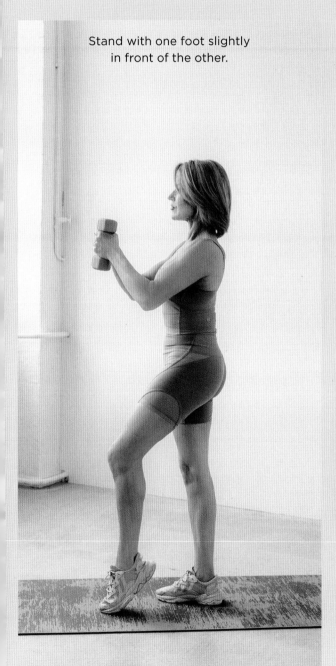

Sink down into the back leg by bending the back knee with the front heel up.

Try not to sink into the hip by keeping the hips as square as possible.

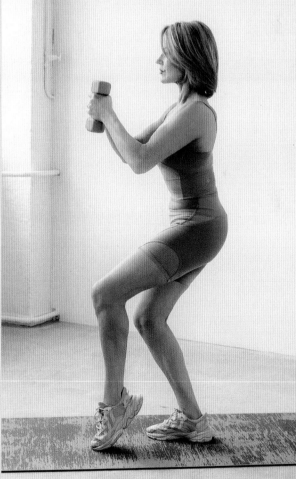

Plank

This is another challenging yoga posture. But keep in mind that you can start on your knees and pull your belly in as you hold the position. Once you get stronger, move your knees further away from your elbows. When you feel ready, lift your knees off the floor and make a long line from your head to your heels. You may only be able to hold for a few counts at first and then just come back to your knees. Each time you do it, spend a few more counts in full plank.

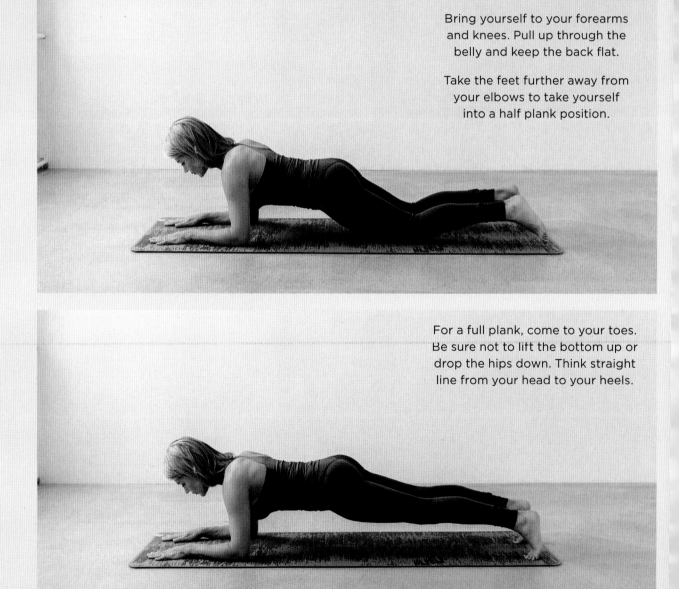

Bring yourself to your forearms and knees. Pull up through the belly and keep the back flat.

Take the feet further away from your elbows to take yourself into a half plank position.

For a full plank, come to your toes. Be sure not to lift the bottom up or drop the hips down. Think straight line from your head to your heels.

What's Next

Once you complete the 4-Week, 15-Minute Menopause Metabolism Fix, you'll have embraced habits that will move you beyond the scope of this program. It's essential to recognize that wellness is a journey without shortcuts. Expecting miraculous change in just four weeks is unrealistic. Yet, I am confident that upon revisiting the quiz from the start of this book, you'll discover a significant reduction in your menopause symptoms.

This progress will fuel your desire to keep going with your newfound practices. Embrace the positivity that comes with knowing things will continuously improve. You'll experience enhanced sleep quality, fewer hot flashes, diminishing belly fat, and an infusion of energy like never before.

To maintain momentum, simply revisit the plan and incorporate daily workouts, aiming for one fifteen-minute session each day. If you're eager to elevate your challenge, consider increasing your weights during certain exercises. It's wise to alternate between your current and heavier weights until you're ready to fully transition to the more challenging set.

For those wishing to pursue this transformative journey alongside me, a further real-time guide is just a QR code away. Scan it to unlock the subsequent phase of your wellness evolution.

Thank you for joining me on this path. I hope to see you soon as you move through and beyond this plan to the next phase of your life! For the follow-up plan and more, visit https://carafitness.co.uk/.

PART
THREE

Eat to Nourish
Your Body

Nutty Green Fruit Smoothie

DAIRY-FREE, GLUTEN-FREE, GRAIN-FREE, HIGH-FIBER, VEGAN, VEGETARIAN

Coconut milk and pea protein powder offer healthy fats and protein, supporting hormonal health during menopause. A frozen banana provides potassium for heart health, while baby spinach delivers magnesium for bones. Strawberries add vitamin C for skin and immune function, and almond butter brings vitamin E and fats to aid in symptom relief. A pinch of sea salt helps with electrolyte balance, making this smoothie a beneficial choice for menopause support.

SERVINGS: 2 • PREP TIME: 5 minutes • COOK TIME: 0 minutes

- 2 cups (475 ml) plain and unsweetened coconut milk (or your choice of plant-based milk)
- 4 scoops (60 g) plain and unsweetened pea protein powder
- 1 medium (4 ounces, or 115 g) frozen banana
- 4 cups (172 g) baby spinach
- 2 cups (290 g) fresh or (298 g) frozen strawberries
- ¼ cup (64 g) raw almond butter
- Pinch sea salt

1 Add all the ingredients into a blender and blend on high speed until very creamy. If you prefer a thinner smoothie, add more milk, ¼ cup (60 ml) at a time, until it has blended to your desired consistency.

2 Serve immediately.

3 Enjoy!

NUTRITION INFO:

Calories: 468
Fat: 21g
Carbs: 40g
Net Carbs: 30g
Fiber: 10g
Protein: 39g

All-the-Berries Smoothie with Cauliflower

DAIRY-FREE, GLUTEN-FREE, GRAIN-FREE, HIGH-FIBER, VEGAN, VEGETARIAN

Coconut milk and pea protein powder provide healthy fats and protein to support hormonal balance in menopause. Avocado, rich in good fats, helps maintain skin health. Baby spinach offers bone-strengthening calcium and magnesium. Berries, including strawberries and cranberries, deliver antioxidants and vitamin C for immune function and skin vitality. Frozen riced cauliflower adds volume without excess calories, aiding in weight management. A pinch of sea salt enhances mineral intake. This combination of ingredients creates a nutrient-dense meal that can help reduce menopause symptoms.

SERVINGS: 2 • PREP TIME: 5 minutes • COOK TIME: 0 minutes

- 2 cups (475 ml) plain and unsweetened coconut milk (or your choice of plant-based milk)
- 4 scoops (60 g) plain and unsweetened pea protein powder
- 1 medium (5.5 ounces, or 150 g) avocado, peeled and pitted
- 4 cups (172 g) baby spinach
- 2 cups (280 g) fresh or (326 g) frozen mixed berries
- 1 cup (145 g) fresh or (149 g) frozen strawberries
- 2 cups (200 g) frozen riced cauliflower
- ¼ cup (33 g) fresh or frozen cranberries
- Pinch sea salt

1 Add all the ingredients into a blender and blend on high speed until very creamy. If you prefer a thinner smoothie, add more milk, ¼ cup (60 ml) at a time, until it has blended to your desired consistency.

2 Serve immediately.

3 Enjoy!

NUTRITION INFO:

Calories: 454
Fat: 15g
Carbs: 46g
Net Carbs: 33g
Fiber: 13g
Protein: 33g

Roasted Carrots with Pistachios and Mint Greek Yogurt

GLUTEN-FREE, GRAIN-FREE, HIGH-FIBER, VEGETARIAN

Chopped carrots, rich in beta-carotene, support eye health and immunity, which can be beneficial during menopause. Avocado oil adds healthy fats for hormone regulation. Garlic provides antioxidants, while optional cumin and cardamom offer digestive and anti-inflammatory benefits. Sea salt and black pepper enhance the dish with essential minerals and a flavor boost. The garnish of lemon zest adds vitamin C, with cilantro or parsley contributing detoxifying properties. Toasted pistachios lend heart-healthy fats and a satisfying crunch.

The accompanying Mint Greek Yogurt, with its probiotics, supports digestive health, and the mint may provide a cooling effect, potentially easing hot flashes. The scallion adds a mild, peppery taste, rounding out a nourishing meal that targets menopause symptoms.

SERVINGS: 6 • PREP TIME: 10 minutes • COOK TIME: 30–35 minutes

Roasted Carrots:

- 12 medium (25.5 ounces, or 720 g) carrots, peeled and chopped
- 2 tablespoons (28 ml) avocado oil
- 2 small (0.5 ounces, or 8 g) garlic cloves, peeled and minced
- 1 teaspoon (6 g) sea salt
- ½ teaspoon (1 g) black pepper
- 1 teaspoon (2 g) ground cumin (optional)
- Sprinkle ground cardamom (optional)

For Garnish:

- Zest from ½ (0.5 ounces, or 13 g) medium fresh lemon
- ¼ cup (15 g) fresh minced cilantro or parsley
- ¼ cup (31 g) toasted pistachios

Mint Greek Yogurt:

- 2 cups (454 g) full-fat plain Greek yogurt
- 1 teaspoon (6 g) sea salt
- Zest from ½ (0.5 ounces, or 13 g) medium fresh lemon
- 5–8 fresh mint leaves, minced
- 1 whole medium (0.5 ounces, or 15 g) scalllon, minced

1 Preheat the oven to 400°F (200°C, or gas mark 6).

2 To prepare the carrots, add the carrots, avocado oil, garlic, sea salt, black pepper, and cumin and cardamom (if using) to a mixing bowl and toss well together.

3 Arrange the carrots on a baking tray lined with parchment paper and roast until very soft and caramelized, 30–35 minutes, tossing at the half-way mark. When done, remove from the oven, garnish with lemon zest, cilantro or parsley, and toasted pistachios.

4 While the carrots are roasting, prepare the Mint Greek Yogurt by adding the Greek yogurt, sea salt, lemon zest, mint, and scallion to a bowl and mixing thoroughly so that everything is combined evenly.

5 Serve the Roasted Carrots with a side of Mint Greek Yogurt, storing any leftovers in the fridge in an airtight container for up to 5 days.

6 Enjoy!

NUTRITION INFO:

Calories: 103
Fat: 7g
Carbs: 7g
Net Carbs: 5g
Fiber: 2g
Protein: 4g

Poppy Seed Protein Pancakes with Raspberry Sauce

GLUTEN-FREE, HIGH-FIBER, HIGH-PROTEIN, LOWER-CARB, VEGETARIAN

Oat flour, derived from oats, offers dietary fiber beneficial for weight management and heart health during menopause, and its B vitamins can aid in mood stabilization. Greek yogurt provides essential calcium and protein, supporting bone health as osteoporosis risks rise during menopause. Eggs, rich in protein and vitamin D, further bolster bone health.

Though almond milk's phytoestrogens are less potent than those in soy milk, it can offer minor relief from menopausal symptoms and if fortified, adds calcium. Raspberries, like other berries, supply antioxidants and vitamins, promoting general health during menopause. Pecans are heart-healthy nuts and contribute beneficial fats and nutrients, crucial for cardiovascular health in menopause.

SERVINGS: 2 • PREP TIME: 10 minutes • COOK TIME: 15–20 minutes

Raspberry Sauce:
- 1 cup (125 g) fresh raspberries
- 1–2 tablespoons (15–28 ml) purified water
- 1 tablespoon (20 g) raw honey or pure maple syrup
- ½ teaspoon (2.5 ml) pure vanilla extract

Pancakes:
- 1 cup (120 g) gluten-free oat flour (If using raw whole oats, pulse the oats in a food processor until you attain a flour consistency.)
- 2 scoops (30 g) plain and unsweetened pea protein powder
- 2 tablespoons (18 g) poppy seeds
- 1 teaspoon (5 g) baking powder
- ½ teaspoon (3 g) baking soda
- ¼ teaspoon (2 g) fine sea salt
- 1 cup (227 g) full-fat plain Greek yogurt
- 2 large (3.5 ounces, or 100 g) eggs
- ¼ cup (60 ml) plain and unsweetened almond milk
- 1 tablespoon (20 g) raw honey or pure maple syrup (optional)
- 1 teaspoon (5 ml) pure vanilla extract
- Coconut oil to grease skillet

For Garnish:
- 1 cup (227 g) 2% plain Greek yogurt
- ¼ (28 g) cup chopped pecans

140

1 Prepare the Raspberry Sauce by adding the raspberries and water in a small saucepan and bringing to a simmer for 5 to 7 minutes, stirring and breaking up the raspberries often. Add the raw honey or maple syrup and pure vanilla extract and simmer, stirring often, for another 2 to 3 minutes. Remove from the heat and set aside.

2 To prepare the pancake batter, combine the oat flour, pea protein powder, poppy seeds, baking powder, baking soda, and sea salt in one bowl and stir together well.

3 Add the Greek yogurt, eggs, almond milk, raw honey or maple syrup (if using), and pure vanilla extract in a separate bowl. Whisk together thoroughly and then add it to the dry ingredients and stir well so that the batter is evenly combined.

4 Heat a large, flat skillet to medium-low heat and melt enough coconut oil on the skillet to grease it well.

5 Pour ¼ cup (60 ml) portions of batter onto the skillet. Let cook for 2 to 3 minutes or until the pancakes begin to bubble and the edges have begun to set. Carefully flip with a spatula and finish cooking for another 1 to 2 minutes on the opposite side.

6 Continue to make additional pancakes until all the batter has been used.

7 Serve with Raspberry Sauce, Greek yogurt, and chopped pecans, storing any leftovers in the fridge in an airtight container for up to 2 days.

8 Enjoy!

Notes about the recipe: Poppy seeds are a wonderful addition to these protein-packed pancakes. Poppy seeds are high in protein, fiber, calcium, magnesium, and zinc and have been known to aid digestion.

NUTRITION INFO:

Calories: 424
Fat: 18g
Carbs: 41g
Net Carbs: 36g
Fiber: 5g
Protein: 26g

Cranberry and Bulgur Wheat Breakfast Bowl

HIGH-FIBER, HIGH-PROTEIN, LOWER-CARB, VEGETARIAN

Bulgur wheat is a whole grain, which is good for heart health. This matters because cardiovascular risks elevate post-menopause due to declining estrogen levels. Its fiber content aids in digestion and weight regulation. Pecans, rich in beneficial fats and nutrients, also enhance cardiovascular and overall health during menopause.

Dried cranberries offer antioxidants and may promote urinary tract health, though one should monitor added sugars. Blueberries, abundant in vitamins, antioxidants, and phytonutrients, support general healthiness and counteract increased oxidative stress in menopause. Cinnamon assists in stabilizing blood sugar, crucial as insulin sensitivity may vary during menopause.

SERVINGS: 2 • PREP TIME: 5 minutes • COOK TIME: 10–12 minutes

Cranberry and Bulgar Wheat:

- 1 cup (180 g) bulgur wheat
- ½ teaspoon (2 g) fine sea salt
- 1 teaspoon (3 g) ground cinnamon
- 2 cups (475 ml) purified water
- ¼ cup (30 g) dried cranberries

For Garnish:

- ½ cup (114 g) full-fat plain Greek yogurt
- ¼ cup (28 g) chopped pecans
- ½ cup (73 g) fresh blueberries

1 In a medium saucepan, combine the bulgur wheat, sea salt, cinnamon, and water. Bring to a boil, reduce the heat to low, cover, and stir in the cranberries. Let it simmer for 10 to 12 minutes or until the bulgur wheat is tender and the liquid is absorbed. Turn off the stove and remove from the heat.

2 Serve with Greek yogurt, chopped pecans, and blueberries, storing any leftovers in the fridge in an airtight container for up to 3 days.

3 Enjoy!

Notes about the recipe : Dried fruit doesn't always have to be consumed dry. Did you know you can rehydrate it by simply soaking or simmering it in water? This breakfast bowl plumps dried cranberries, which add delicious, tart flavor to an ancient grain.

NUTRITION INFO:

Calories: 479
Fat: 12g
Carbs: 73g
Net Carbs: 65g
Fiber: 8g
Protein: 16g

Flaxseed Porridge with Raspberries and Hazelnut Butter

DAIRY-FREE, GLUTEN-FREE, VEGAN, VEGETARIAN

Steel-cut oats provide dietary fiber, which is beneficial in terms of weight management and heart health and contain B vitamins that help manage mood and stress during menopause. Ground flaxseed contains phyto-estrogens like lignans, which may balance hormones, potentially easing menopausal symptoms. Flaxseeds also offer heart-healthy omega-3 fatty acids. Pea protein powder aids in preserving muscle mass, which can diminish with age, and assists in weight regulation. Raspberries, rich in antioxidants, bolster overall health. Hazelnut butter and chopped hazelnuts, abundant in healthy fats, vitamins, and minerals, enhance cardio-vascular health, particularly crucial during menopause.

SERVINGS: 2 • PREP TIME: 5 minutes • COOK TIME: 10 minutes

BREAKFAST/BRUNCH

Flaxseed Porridge:

- 2 cups (475 ml) almond milk (or your choice of plant-based milk)
- 1 cup (176 g) raw gluten-free steel-cut oats
- 1 tablespoon (7 g) ground flaxseed
- Pinch sea salt
- 2 scoops (30 g) plain pea protein powder
- ¼ cup (31 g) fresh raspberries, chopped
- 2 tablespoons (32 g) hazelnut butter

For Garnish:

- ¼ cup (31 g) fresh raspberries
- 2 tablespoons (29 g) chopped hazelnuts

1 Add the almond milk, steel-cut oats, ground flaxseed, and sea salt to a saucepan and bring to a boil. Once boiling, reduce heat to a simmer and stir often for 5 to 8 minutes.

2 Turn off the heat and stir in the plain pea protein powder, raspberries, and hazelnut butter.

3 Remove from the heat and serve with additional raspberries and chopped hazelnuts, storing any leftovers in an airtight container in the fridge for up to 3 days.

4 Enjoy!

Notes about the recipe: This fiber-packed porridge is a great way to start the day! Make a big batch of this to enjoy throughout the week. For even more protein, serve this with 1–2 soft-boiled eggs.

NUTRITION INFO:

Calories: 446
Fat: 20g
Carbs: 45g
Net Carbs: 35g
Fiber: 10g
Protein: 24g

Avocado and Spinach Scramble

GLUTEN-FREE, GRAIN-FREE, LOWER-CARB, VEGETARIAN

Avocados and avocado oil are rich in monounsaturated fats, promoting cardiovascular health, which is especially critical during menopause when heart risk escalates. Avocados also offer fiber, potassium, and various vitamins. Coconut oil, containing medium-chain triglycerides, can provide health perks like energy metabolism, though since it contains saturated fat, use it in moderation. Turmeric, rich in anti-inflammatory curcumin, can be beneficial due to increased inflammation concerns during menopause.

SERVINGS: 2 • PREP TIME: 5 minutes • COOK TIME: 10 minutes

Scramble:

- 1 teaspoon (5 g) avocado or coconut oil
- 2 tablespoons (20 g) peeled and minced red onion
- 1 small (0.1 ounces, or 4 g) garlic clove, peeled and minced
- ¼ medium (1.5 ounces, or 38 g) red bell pepper, seeded and diced
- ½ teaspoon (3 g) sea salt
- ¼ teaspoon (0.5 g) black pepper
- 1 teaspoon (2 g) ground turmeric
- 1 cup (43 g) baby spinach
- 4 large (7 ounces, or 200 g) eggs
- ½ cup (75 g) cherry tomatoes, halved
- 1 medium (5.5 ounces, or 150 g) avocado, peeled and diced

For Garnish:

- 1 cup (227 g) full-fat plain Greek yogurt

NUTRITION INFO:

Calories: 475
Fat: 34g
Carbs: 14g
Net Carbs: 8g
Fiber: 6g
Protein: 30g

1 Add the avocado or coconut oil to a large sauté pan and set the heat to medium-low.

2 When the pan is hot, add the red onion and garlic and sauté, stirring often, until soft, about 3 minutes. Add the red bell pepper and season with sea salt, black pepper, and turmeric. Sauté, stirring often until soft, about 3 minutes.

3 Add the baby spinach and stir until it's wilted.

4 Crack the eggs into the pan and quickly stir into the veggies, scraping up the bottom and sides of the pan until the eggs are fully cooked, 1 to 2 minutes.

5 Turn off the heat and gently stir in the cherry tomatoes and avocado.

6 Serve immediately, with a side of Greek yogurt, storing any leftovers in an airtight container in the fridge for up to 2 days.

7 Enjoy!

Spiced Oats with Sliced Peaches and Pistachios

DAIRY-FREE, GLUTEN-FREE, HIGH-FIBER, VEGAN, VEGETARIAN

Almond milk provides a lactose-free base, rich in calcium and vitamin E, essential for skin and bone health, especially during menopause. Raw steel-cut oats are whole grains that support heart health and offer sustained energy. Chia seeds are rich in omega-3 fatty acids, vital for cognitive function and mood stabilization. The garnish combines almond butter's healthy fats, peaches' vitamins and fiber, and pistachios' protein and antioxidants.

SERVINGS: 2 • PREP TIME: 5 minutes • COOK TIME: 5 minutes

Oats:

- 2 cups (475 ml) almond milk (or your choice of plant-based milk)
- 1 cup (176 g) raw gluten-free steel-cut oats
- 2 tablespoons (26 g) chia seeds
- Pinch sea salt
- 1 teaspoon (3 g) ground cinnamon
- ½ teaspoon (1 g) ground cardamom
- Pinch ground nutmeg
- Pinch ground cloves

For Garnish:

- 2 tablespoons (32 g) raw almond butter (or nut butter of choice)
- 2 medium (300 g) fresh peaches, pitted and sliced
- 2 tablespoons (14 g) chopped pistachios
- 4–5 fresh mint leaves, minced

1 Add the almond milk, steel-cut oats, chia seeds, and sea salt to a saucepan and bring to a boil. Once boiling, reduce heat to a simmer and stir often for about 5 minutes.

2 Turn off the heat and stir in the cinnamon, cardamom, nutmeg, and cloves.

3 Remove from the heat and serve, garnishing with raw almond butter, peach slices, pistachios, and mint, storing any leftovers in an airtight container in the fridge for up to 3 days.

4 Enjoy!

Notes about the recipe: Peaches offer a variety of vitamins and minerals, but if you don't have access to them, simply replace them with another serving of fresh fruit!

NUTRITION INFO:

Calories: 451
Fat: 21g
Carbs: 55g
Net Carbs: 40g
Fiber: 15g
Protein: 15g

Chickpea Flour Pancakes with Lemony Tahini Sauce and a Side Salad

GLUTEN-FREE, HIGH-PROTEIN, HIGH-FIBER, LOWER-CARB, VEGETARIAN

Chickpea flour serves as a protein-packed base, supporting muscle mass and metabolism during menopause. Turmeric, with its anti-inflammatory properties, can help alleviate joint discomfort that some women experience. Nutritional yeast provides B vitamins, crucial for energy and mood balance. Fresh herbs like parsley, dill, and scallion add flavor and vital micronutrients.

Almond milk offers a dairy-free calcium source, supporting bone health. Coconut oil's medium-chain triglycerides can boost metabolism. The Lemon Tahini Sauce introduces healthy fats and a tangy flavor, while the baby kale, asparagus, radishes, and avocado in the Side Salad provide fiber, vitamins, and minerals essential for overall wellness during menopause.

SERVINGS: 2 • PREP TIME: 15 minutes • COOK TIME: 20 minutes

Lemon Tahini Sauce:
- ¼ cup (60 g) tahini
- ¼ cup (60 ml) purified water
- 1 tablespoon (15 ml) fresh lemon juice
- Zest from ½ medium (0.5 ounces, or 13 g) fresh lemon
- ¼ teaspoon (2 g) fine sea salt

Side Salad:
- 2 teaspoons (10 ml) olive oil
- ¼ teaspoon (2 g) fine sea salt
- 2 cups (85 g) baby kale
- 1 cup (134 g) chopped fresh asparagus, tough ends removed
- ½ cup (58 g) diced radishes, ends removed
- ½ medium (3 ounces, or 75 g) avocado, peeled and diced

Pancakes:
- 1 cup (120 g) chickpea flour
- 1 teaspoon (2 g) ground turmeric
- 1 tablespoon (4 g) nutritional yeast
- ¼ teaspoon (2 g) fine sea salt
- 1 cup (235 ml) plain and unsweetened almond milk
- ¼ cup (15 g) minced fresh parsley
- ¼ cup (16 g) minced fresh dill
- 1 whole medium (0.5 ounces, or 15 g) scallion, minced
- Coconut oil or grass-fed butter to grease skillet

1 Prepare the Lemon Tahini Sauce by adding the tahini, water, lemon juice, lemon zest, and sea salt in a bowl. Whisk until everything is well combined and very creamy. Set aside.

2 Prepare the side salad by adding the olive oil and sea salt to a large mixing bowl. Add the baby kale, asparagus, radishes, and avocado to the bowl and gently toss until everything is evenly coated in the olive oil mixture. Set aside.

3 To prepare the Pancake batter, combine the chickpea flour, turmeric, nutritional yeast, and sea salt in one bowl and stir together well.

4 Add the almond milk, half of the parsley, dill, and scallion to the dry ingredients and stir well so that the batter is evenly combined.

5 Heat a large, flat skillet to medium-low heat and melt enough coconut oil or butter on the skillet to grease it well.

6 Pour ¼ cup (60 ml) portions of batter onto the skillet. Let cook for 1 to 2 minutes or until the pancakes become golden and the edges have set. Carefully flip with a spatula and finish cooking for another 1 minute on the opposite side.

7 Continue to make additional pancakes until all the batter has been used.

8 Serve with the Lemon Tahini Sauce, the remaining minced parsley, dill, and scallion, and a side salad, storing any leftovers in the fridge in an airtight container for up to 2 days.

9 Enjoy!

Notes about the recipe: Chickpea flour is naturally high in protein, making it an excellent option to use in these savory herbed pancakes. Adding a Side Salad ensures you get plenty of vitamins and minerals in every bite of this recipe, which can be had for breakfast, lunch, or dinner!

NUTRITION INFO:

Calories: 525
Fat: 30g
Carbs: 46g
Net Carbs: 33g
Fiber: 13g
Protein: 21g

Butternut Egg Bake with Herbs and Sunflower Seeds

DAIRY-FREE, GLUTEN-FREE, HIGH-FIBER, VEGETARIAN

Avocado oil aids hormonal balance during menopause, while butternut squash's nutrients support skin hydration. Baby spinach boosts bone health, crucial during menopausal changes. Eggs offer protein for tissue repair, and almond milk combats menopausal dryness. Nutritional yeast provides energy-boosting B vitamins. Fresh herbs and garlic help reduce inflammation, while sunflower seeds support mood and thyroid health. The avocado garnish offers essential fats for hormone production. This dish is both delicious and tailored for menopausal health.

SERVINGS: 4 • PREP TIME: 10 minutes • COOK TIME: 25 minutes

- 2 tablespoons (28 ml) avocado oil
- 2 cups (340g) cubed butternut squash
- 2 teaspoons (12 g) sea salt, divided
- 1 teaspoon (2 g) black pepper, divided
- 4 cups (172 g) baby spinach, chopped
- 12 large (21 ounces, or 600 g) eggs
- ½ cup (120 ml) plain and unsweetened almond milk
- 1 tablespoon (6 g) fresh lemon zest
- 2 tablespoons (8 g) nutritional yeast
- 1 small (0.1 ounces, or 4 g) garlic clove, peeled and minced

For Garnish:
- ¼ cup (6 g) fresh basil leaves
- ¼ cup (15 g) minced fresh parsley
- ¼ cup (36 g) sunflower seeds

For Serving:
- 2 medium (11 ounces, or 300 g) avocados, peeled and sliced

1 Preheat the oven to 400°F (200°C, or gas mark 6) and line an 8 x 8-inch (20 x 20 cm) oven-safe baking dish with parchment paper.

2 Add avocado oil to a skillet set to medium heat.

3 Add the butternut squash and season with 1 teaspoon (6 g) sea salt and ½ teaspoon (1 g) black pepper. Sauté until soft, about 5 minutes. Add the baby spinach and continue to sauté until the spinach has wilted, about 3 minutes. Remove from the heat and set aside.

4 Crack the eggs into a large mixing bowl and whisk well. Add the almond milk and mix.

5 Season the whisked eggs with the remaining 1 teaspoon (6 g) sea salt and ½ teaspoon (1 g) black pepper, lemon zest, nutritional yeast, and garlic and mix thoroughly.

6 Spread the sautéed butternut squash and wilted baby spinach into the baking dish lined with parchment paper in an even layer. Pour the egg mixture over the veggies.

7 Bake in the oven for 18 to 22 minutes. It will be done when the eggs are set and no longer runny.

8 Remove from the oven, garnish with the basil and parsley, and sprinkle with sunflower seeds.

9 Let cool for a few minutes before slicing into 4 large squares.

10 Serve with sliced avocado, storing any leftovers in the fridge in an airtight container for up to 3 days.

11 Enjoy!

Notes about the recipe: Starting the day with protein ensures you feel satisfied to take on the day's activities. Adding healthy fats, such as avocado, helps your body absorb the vitamins and minerals in this recipe.

NUTRITION INFO:

Calories: 447
Fat: 33g
Carbs: 18g
Net Carbs: 10g
Fiber: 8g
Protein: 23g

Coconut Yogurt with Berries and Muesli

DAIRY-FREE, GLUTEN-FREE, HIGH-FIBER, VEGAN, VEGETARIAN

The probiotics in coconut yogurt aid gut health and are excellent for helping to manage menopausal symptoms. The berries provide antioxidants, vital during hormonal changes. Raw steel-cut oats ensure lasting energy to keep you going throughout the morning. Hemp seeds, rich in omega fatty acids, support brain health, crucial during menopause. Hazelnuts and cacao nibs offer healthy fats and mood-boosting properties, respectively, which help to manage mood swings. This dish is tailored for flavor and menopause symptom relief.

SERVINGS: 2 • PREP TIME: 10 minutes • COOK TIME: 0 minutes

Yogurt and Fruit:
- 1 teaspoon (4 g) vanilla bean powder
- 2 cups (454 g) plain coconut yogurt
- ¼ cup (39 g) fresh cherries, pitted and halved
- ¼ cup (31 g) fresh raspberries, halved
- ¼ cup (36 g) fresh blackberries, halved
- ¼ cup (36 g) fresh blueberries

Muesli:
- ½ cup (88 g) raw gluten-free steel-cut oats
- 2 tablespoons (18 g) unsweetened raisins
- 2 tablespoons (18 g) hemp seeds
- 2 tablespoons (16 g) raw or toasted hazelnuts, chopped
- 2 tablespoons (15 g) raw cacao nibs

1 Stir the vanilla bean powder into the coconut yogurt.

2 Top the yogurt with the cherriesraspberries, blackberries, and blueberries.

3 Prepare the muesli by mixing the steel-cut oats, raisins, hemp seeds, hazelnuts, and cacao nibs together. Sprinkle over the yogurt and fruit.

4 Serve, storing any leftovers in an airtight container in the fridge for up to 3 days.

5 Enjoy!

Notes about the recipe: Coconut yogurt is a wonderful source of probiotics. If you tolerate dairy well, you can use 2% plain Greek yogurt as another option. It will still offer probiotics, and its high protein will help you stay satisfied in between meals.

NUTRITION INFO:

Calories: 429
Fat: 18g
Carbs: 61g
Net Carbs: 48g
Fiber: 13g
Protein: 8g

Toast with Avocado Mash and a Side of Cheesy Scramble

HIGH-FIBER, VEGETARIAN

Sourdough bread offers easier digestion with beneficial prebiotics. Coconut oil and grass-fed butter contribute healthy fats for hormone production. Avocado in the mash provides heart-healthy fats and fiber, with red pepper flakes potentially boosting metabolism. The eggs in the scramble deliver protein and choline for muscle and brain health, while leafy greens like arugula supply essential calcium and iron for bone strength. Cheese adds extra calcium and protein, supporting overall menopause health.

SERVINGS: 2 • PREP TIME: 5 minutes • COOK TIME: 10 minutes

Avocado Mash:

- 1 medium (5.5 ounces, or 150 g) avocado, peeled and mashed gently with a fork
- ½ teaspoon (3 g) sea salt
- ½ teaspoon (0.5 g) dried red pepper flakes

Cheesy Scramble:

- 1 teaspoon (5 g) avocado or coconut oil
- 4 large (7 ounces, or 200 g) eggs
- ½ teaspoon (3 g) sea salt
- ¼ teaspoon (0.5 g) black pepper
- 2 cups (40 g) arugula or another leafy green, chopped
- 1 ounce (28 g) of your favorite cheese such as shredded extra-sharp cheddar, crumbled goat, or crumbled feta

Toast:

- 2 slices of fresh sourdough bread (Look for bread with minimal ingredients, such as only wheat, water, and salt.)
- 2 teaspoons (10 g) coconut oil or grass-fed butter

1 For the Avocado Mash, stir the sea salt and red pepper flakes into the mashed avocado.

2 Toast the sourdough and spread it with coconut oil or grass-fed butter. Top the toast with the Avocado Mash.

3 Add the avocado or coconut oil to a large sauté pan and set the heat to medium-low. When the pan is hot, crack the eggs into the pan, season with sea salt and black pepper, and quickly stir with a spatula, breaking up the yolks, scraping up the bottom and sides of the pan until the eggs are fully cooked, 1 to 2 minutes. Stir in the arugula and let it wilt.

4 Turn off the heat and top with your choice of cheese. Give the eggs a few tosses.

5 Serve immediately.

6 Enjoy!

NUTRITION INFO:

Calories: 495
Fat: 32g
Carbs: 31g
Net Carbs: 25g
Fiber: 6g
Protein: 21g

Spelt Porridge with Caramelized Banana and Pecans

DAIRY-FREE, HIGH-FIBER, VEGAN, VEGETARIAN

Ground flaxseed adds lignans, which may help balance hormones and manage menopause symptoms. Topped with Greek yogurt for probiotics and protein, and pecans for a magnesium boost, this meal is both wholesome and menopause-friendly.

SERVINGS: 2 • PREP TIME: 10 minutes • COOK TIME: 20 minutes

Spelt Porridge:
- 1 cup (120 g) cracked spelt
- 2 cups (475 ml) purified water
- 1 cup (235 ml) plain and unsweetened almond milk (or your choice of plant-based milk)
- Pinch sea salt
- 1 tablespoon (7 g) ground flaxseed

Caramelized Banana:
- 1 teaspoon (5 g) coconut oil
- 2 medium (8 ounces, or 230 g) bananas, peeled and sliced in ½-inch (1.3 cm) rounds
- Pinch sea salt
- 1 tablespoon (8 g) ground cinnamon

For Garnish:
- ½ Caramelized Banana recipe
- 2 tablespoons (14 g) chopped pecans
- ½ cup (114 g) full-fat plain Greek yogurt (Omit to keep this recipe Vegan and Dairy-Free.)

NUTRITION INFO:
Calories: 497
Fat: 14g
Carbs: 79g
Net Carbs: 66g
Fiber: 13g
Protein: 19g

1 Add the cracked spelt, water, and almond milk to a saucepan, bring to a boil, and then reduce to a simmer until the spelt is tender, about 20 minutes. Stir in the sea salt and ground flaxseed.

2 While the spelt is simmering, prepare your Caramelized Bananas. Add coconut oil to a skillet and bring to medium-low heat. Add the sliced bananas and season with sea salt and cinnamon, tossing together until the bananas are coated in cinnamon.

3 Sauté on low heat until the bananas are soft and fragrant, about 5 minutes. Turn off the heat.

4 When the spelt is done cooking, turn off the heat and stir in half of the Caramelized Bananas until well combined.

5 Top your porridge with the remaining Caramelized Bananas and chopped pecans and a dollop of Greek yogurt (if using).

6 Serve, storing any leftovers in the fridge in an airtight container for up to 3 days.

7 Enjoy!

Good Morning Breakfast Burrito

HIGH-FIBER, VEGETARIAN

Avocado or coconut oil provides healthy fats, crucial for menopausal hormonal health. Eggs are a high-quality protein source, helping to maintain muscle mass during menopause. Baby spinach offers iron and calcium, key for bone strength, which is often compromised during menopause. The capsaicin in red pepper flakes may help boost metabolism.

SERVINGS: 2 • PREP TIME: 5 minutes • COOK TIME: 10 minutes

Scramble:

- 1 teaspoon (5 g) avocado or coconut oil
- 6 large (11 ounces, or 300 g) eggs
- ½ teaspoon (3 g) sea salt
- ¼ teaspoon (0.5 g) black pepper
- 2 cups (86 g) baby spinach or another leafy green, chopped
- ½ medium (75 g) avocado, peeled and diced
- ½ teaspoon (0.5 g) dried red pepper flakes
- 1 ounce (28 g) crumbled goat or crumbled feta cheese
- 2 whole grain tortillas

For Garnish (Optional):

- Hot sauce
- Salsa
- Fresh cilantro, minced

1 Add the avocado or coconut oil to a large sauté pan and set the heat to medium-low.

2 When the pan is hot, crack the eggs into the pan, season with sea salt and black pepper, and quickly stir with a spatula, breaking up the yolks, scraping up the bottom sides of the pan until the eggs are fully cooked, 1 to 2 minutes. Stir in the baby spinach and let it wilt. Add the avocado and red pepper flakes and gently combine it into the scramble.

3 Turn off the heat and top with your choice of cheese, letting it melt onto the eggs. Give the eggs a few quick tosses, so that the cheese spreads throughout the eggs.

4 Fill each tortilla with the scramble and roll up as a burrito.

5 Serve immediately, with the optional hot sauce, salsa, and cilantro.

6 Enjoy!

BREAKFAST/BRUNCH

NUTRITION INFO:

Calories: 484
Fat: 31g
Carbs: 29g
Net Carbs: 23g
Fiber: 6g
Protein: 24g

Salmon Salad with Green Beans and Avocado

DAIRY-FREE, GLUTEN-FREE, HIGH-FIBER, HIGH-PROTEIN, LOWER-CARB

Green beans and wild-caught salmon, rich in omega-3s, support hormonal balance during menopause. The zesty lemon and seasonings enhance mood and energy. Arugula, with its peppery flavor, aids in bone health, crucial during menopause. The tangy dressing, combined with the sharpness of red onion, helps manage menopausal symptoms. Pumpkin seeds, loaded with magnesium and zinc, address sleep issues common in menopause. Avocado's creaminess offers healthy fats for overall contentment. This dish is tailored for flavor and easing menopausal discomforts.

SERVINGS: 2 • PREP TIME: 10 minutes • COOK TIME: 15–20 minutes

Green Beans:
- 2 cups (475 ml) purified water
- ½ pound (225 g) green beans, ends removed

Salmon:
- ½ pound (225 g) wild-caught salmon fillets (skin on)
- 1 tablespoon (15 ml) fresh lemon juice
- 1 teaspoon (6 g) sea salt
- ½ teaspoon (1 g) black pepper
- 2 teaspoons (4 g) dried Italian seasoning

Salad:
- 2 tablespoons (28 ml) olive oil
- 1 tablespoon (15 ml) raw apple cider vinegar
- 1 teaspoon (5 g) stone-ground mustard
- 2 tablespoons (20 g) peeled and minced red onion
- Zest from ½ medium (0.5 ounces, or 13 g) fresh lemon
- 1 teaspoon (6 g) sea salt
- ½ teaspoon (1 g) black pepper
- 1 teaspoon (2 g) dried Italian seasoning
- ¼ cup (15 g) minced fresh parsley
- 4 cups (80 g) arugula, chopped
- 2 tablespoons (17 g) raw pumpkin seeds
- ½ medium (75 g) avocado, peeled and diced

1 Add water to a medium saucepan and arrange a steamer basket filled with the trimmed green beans inside the pan. Bring to high heat and once boiling, reduce the heat to a simmer and steam the green beans until tender, about 10 minutes. Once done, transfer to a bowl filled with ice water to stop the green beans from further cooking. When the green beans are very cool, remove from the ice bath and pat dry. Set aside.

2 Preheat the oven to 400°F (200°C, or gas mark 6). Line a baking tray with parchment paper and pat the salmon dry with a paper towel. Squeeze lemon juice over each salmon fillet and season with sea salt, black pepper, and Italian seasoning. Bake in the oven until the salmon is light pink in color and flakes easily with a fork, 15 to 20 minutes. Remove from the oven and set aside. When cool enough to touch, remove the skin and discard.

3 Add the olive oil, apple cider vinegar, stone-ground mustard, red onion, lemon zest, sea salt, black pepper, Italian seasoning, parsley, arugula, pumpkin seeds, and avocado to a large mixing bowl and combine well.

4 Chop the steamed green beans and baked salmon, add to the salad bowl, and gently toss together until everything is well combined.

5 Serve, storing any leftovers in the fridge in an airtight container for up to 2 days.

6 Enjoy!

Notes about the recipe: This dish is high in protein, fiber, and healthy fats. Salmon is a great source of omega-3 fatty acids, which contribute to better mood, skin, and joint health.

NUTRITION INFO:

Calories: 483
Fat: 33g
Carbs: 17g
Net Carbs: 10g
Fiber: 7g
Protein: 34g

Greek Salad with Tempeh and Chickpeas

DAIRY-FREE, HIGH-FIBER, HIGH-PROTEIN, VEGETARIAN, VEGAN

Tempeh, a plant-based protein, supports hormone regulation during menopause. The Mediterranean-inspired dressing, with olive oil and red wine vinegar, offers heart health benefits vital for menopausal women. The mix of spinach, cucumber, and tomatoes provides essential nutrients that support bone health. Chickpeas add fiber, aiding in digestive health during menopause, and avocado's healthy fats support stamina.

SERVINGS: 2 • PREP TIME: 10 minutes • COOK TIME: 15–20 minutes

Tempeh:
- 1 tablespoon (15 ml) olive oil
- 4 ounces (115 g) tempeh, crumbled
- 1 teaspoon (6 g) sea salt
- ½ teaspoon (1 g) black pepper
- 2 teaspoons (2 g) dried oregano

Salad:
- 2 tablespoons (28 ml) olive oil
- 1 tablespoon (15 ml) red wine vinegar
- 2 tablespoons (20 g) peeled and minced red onion
- Zest from ½ medium (0.5 ounces, or 13 g) fresh lemon
- 1 teaspoon (6 g) sea salt
- ½ teaspoon (1 g) black pepper
- 1 teaspoon (1 g) dried oregano
- ¼ cup (15 g) minced fresh parsley
- 4 fresh mint leaves, minced
- 1 medium (0.5 ounces, or 15 g) scallion (green parts only), minced
- 1 large (11 ounces, or 301 g) cucumber, seeded and diced
- 1 cup (150 g) cherry tomatoes, halved
- 4 cups (172 g) baby spinach, chopped
- ½ cup (82 g) cooked chickpeas
- ½ medium (3 ounces, or 75 g) avocado, peeled and diced

1 Prepare the tempeh by adding the olive oil, crumbled tempeh, sea salt, black pepper, and oregano to a mixing bowl and toss together very well. Heat a cast-iron skillet or frying pan to medium heat. When hot, pour the tempeh mixture into the pan and allow to heat and sear, moving around with a spatula, until it begins to brown, 5 to 7 minutes. Turn off the heat and set aside to cool.

2 Add the olive oil, red wine vinegar, red onion, lemon zest, sea salt, black pepper, oregano, parsley, mint, and scallion and whisk well. Add the cucumber, cherry tomatoes, baby spinach, chickpeas, and avocado to a large mixing bowl and combine well. Add the cooked and cooled tempeh and mix well again so that everything is evenly combined.

3 Serve, storing any leftovers in the fridge in an airtight container for up to 3 days.

4 Enjoy!

NUTRITION INFO:

Calories: 494
Fat: 34g
Carbs: 40g
Net Carbs: 28g
Fiber: 12g
Protein: 18g

Chicken Salad with Tomato and Watermelon

DAIRY-FREE, GLUTEN-FREE, HIGH-FIBER, HIGH-PROTEIN, LOWER-CARB

Olive oil and red wine vinegar in this dressing supports cardiovascular health, especially important during menopause. Lime's zesty touch can uplift mood, counteracting menopause-induced mood swings. The herbs—parsley, mint, and basil—offer potential cooling effects for hot flashes. Chicken provides protein, aiding in muscle retention, a concern during menopause.

SERVINGS: 2 • PREP TIME: 10 minutes • COOK TIME: 0 minutes

- 2 tablespoons (28 ml) olive oil
- 1 tablespoon (15 ml) red wine vinegar
- 2 tablespoons (20 g) peeled and minced red onion
- 1 tablespoon (15 ml) fresh lime juice
- Zest from ½ medium (0.5 ounces, or 11 g) fresh lime
- 1 teaspoon (6 g) sea salt
- ½ teaspoon (1 g) black pepper
- ¼ cup (15 g) minced fresh parsley
- 4 fresh mint leaves, minced
- ¼ cup (12 g) minced fresh basil leaves
- ½ pound (225 g) leftover cooked boneless and skinless chicken breast, shredded
- 2 cups (300 g) cubed watermelon
- 2 cups (300 g) cherry
- tomatoes, halved
- 1 large (11 ounces, or 301 g) cucumber, seeded and diced
- 4 cups (220 g) mixed lettuce, chopped
- 2 tablespoons (18 g) raw sunflower seeds
- ½ medium (75 g) avocado, peeled and diced

1 Add the olive oil, red wine vinegar, red onion, lime juice, lime zest, sea salt, black pepper, parsley, mint, and basil to a large mixing bowl and whisk until everything is well combined.

2 Add the shredded chicken breast and toss in the vinaigrette.

3 Add the watermelon, cherry tomatoes, cucumber, mixed lettuce, sunflower seeds, and avocado to a large mixing bowl and gently toss until everything is combined.

4 Serve the chicken mixture over the salad, storing any leftovers in the fridge in an airtight container for up to 2 days.

5 Enjoy!

NUTRITION INFO:

Calories: 459
Fat: 27g
Carbs: 18g
Net Carbs: 13g
Fiber: 5g
Protein: 39g

LUNCH

Roasted Butternut, Apple, Ginger, and Squash Soup

DAIRY-FREE, GLUTEN-FREE, HIGH-FIBER, HIGH-PROTEIN, VEGETARIAN

Coconut oil and full-fat coconut milk offer healthy fats that support hormonal balance during menopause. Antioxidants in red onions, garlic, and red bell peppers combat inflammation, which is often heightened during menopause. Butternut squash and apples provide fiber, stabilizing energy levels. Spices like cumin and ginger have anti-inflammatory and digestive benefits. Silken tofu is crucial for bone health, addressing menopause-related bone density decline. Leafy greens ensure essential vitamin intake, while olive oil's monounsaturated fats further assist in hormonal regulation. You'll find that incorporating these ingredients can help mitigate a variety of menopausal symptoms.

SERVINGS: 4 • PREP TIME: 15 minutes • COOK TIME: 60 minutes

- 2 tablespoons (28 g) coconut oil, melted
- 1 medium (5.5 ounces, or 150 g) red onion, peeled and chopped
- 4 small (1 ounce, or 16 g) garlic cloves, peeled and minced
- 4 cups (680 g) cubed butternut squash
- 1 medium (5.5 ounces, or 150 g) apple (any variety), cored and chopped
- 1 medium (5.5 ounces, or 150 g) red bell pepper, seeded and chopped
- 2 medium (4 ounces, or 120 g) carrots chopped, tops removed

- 2 teaspoons (12 g) fine sea salt
- ½ teaspoon (1 g) black pepper
- 1 teaspoon (2 g) ground cumin
- 1 teaspoon (2 g) smoked paprika
- 1 teaspoon (1 g) dried red pepper flakes
- Pinch ground nutmeg
- 4 cups (960 ml) vegetable stock, plus 1–2 cups (235–475 ml) as needed
- 1 can (14 ounces, or 390 ml) full-fat coconut milk
- 2 pounds (910 g) silken tofu, cubed
- 1 teaspoon (2 g) peeled and minced fresh ginger

For Garnish:
- Microgreens or finely chopped leafy greens (spinach, kale, or swiss chard)
- Crumbled feta cheese (Omit to keep this recipe vegan.)
- Toasted chopped pecans (Omit to keep this recipe nut-free.)
- Drizzle olive oil
- Additional sea salt and black pepper

1 Preheat your oven to 400°F (200°C, or gas mark 6).

2 Add the melted coconut oil, red onion, garlic, butternut squash, apple, red bell pepper, carrot, sea salt, black pepper, cumin, smoked paprika, red pepper flakes, and pinch of nutmeg to a large bowl and toss well until everything is well combined.

3 Spread as an even layer on a baking tray lined with parchment paper.

4 Place in the oven and roast until everything is soft and has begun to caramelize, about 45 minutes. Toss once or twice while roasting.

5 Remove from the oven and let cool for a few minutes. Transfer everything on the baking sheet into a blender, scraping down the pan to ensure you get all the drippings and bits off the baking sheet.

6 Add the vegetable stock, canned coconut milk, silken tofu, and ginger to the blender and secure with its lid. Blend on high speed until everything is very creamy. If your soup is too thick for your preference, add 1 cup (235 ml) of vegetable stock at a time and continue blending until it has reached the consistency of your preference. Taste-test the soup and season with additional sea salt and black pepper if desired.

7 Serve with garnishes, storing any leftovers in the fridge in an airtight container for up to 5 days.

8 Enjoy!

LUNCH

Notes about the recipe: A creamy soup is a wonderful dish to serve or reheat for lunch. Enjoy it just as is or with garnishes and a piece of fresh sourdough bread, a side of steamed rice, or over a bowl of creamy polenta.

NUTRITION INFO WITHOUT GARNISHES:

Calories: 499
Fat: 30g
Carbs: 39g
Net Carbs: 31g
Fiber: 8g
Protein: 20g

Quinoa and Black Bean Salad with Celery Seed Vinaigrette

HIGH-PROTEIN, HIGH-FIBER, VEGETARIAN

Quinoa provides essential amino acids and magnesium, which can help alleviate mood swings and muscle cramps related to menopause. The olive oil in the vinaigrette, rich in monounsaturated fats, can aid in hormonal balance. Cucumbers are high in water content and support hydration, crucial during menopause when dry skin can be an issue.

The lycopene in cherry tomatoes supports heart health, dinosaur kale provides calcium and vitamin K for bone health, and black beans contribute protein and fiber, which stabilize energy levels. Pumpkin seeds are rich in magnesium and zinc, helping with sleep quality and mood. Avocados offer healthy fats and fiber, further assisting with hormonal balance. Finally, Greek yogurt provides probiotics that promote a healthy gut, which can impact overall well-being during menopause. All these foods help to holistically address various menopausal symptoms.

SERVINGS: 4 • PREP TIME: 15 minutes • COOK TIME: 15–20 minutes

- ¼ cup (34 g) raw pumpkin seeds
- 1 cup (173 g) quinoa
- 2 cups (475 ml) purified water or low-sodium vegetable stock
- 2 tablespoons (28 ml) olive oil
- 1 tablespoon (15 ml) red wine vinegar
- 1 teaspoon (7 g) raw honey or pure maple syrup (Use maple syrup to keep this recipe vegan.)
- 1 teaspoon (6 g) sea salt

- ½ teaspoon (1 g) black pepper
- ½ teaspoon (1 g) celery seed
- 1 teaspoon (5 g) stone-ground or Dijon mustard
- 1 large (11 ounces, or 301 g) cucumber, seeded and diced
- 1 cup (150 g) cherry tomatoes, halved
- 4 cups (268 g) dinosaur (lacinato) kale, stems removed
- 15 ounces (425 g) cooked black beans, rinsed
- 1 medium (5.5 ounces, or 150 g) avocado, peeled and diced

For Garnish (Optional):
- Drizzle of olive oil
- Spoonful of crumbled feta cheese (Omit to keep this recipe dairy-free and vegan.)
- A big scoop of 2% plain Greek yogurt (Omit to keep this recipe dairy-free and vegan.)

1 To toast the pumpkin seeds, preheat the oven to 350°F (180°C, or gas mark 4). Arrange the pumpkin seeds on a baking tray lined with parchment paper. Toast in the oven for 3 to 5 minutes or until they begin to pop and get golden in color. Remove from the oven and pour into a bowl to cool.

2 In a medium saucepan, combine the quinoa and water or stock. Bring to a boil, reduce the heat to low, cover, and let it simmer for 15 to 20 minutes or until the quinoa is cooked and the liquid is absorbed.

3 Add the olive oil, red wine vinegar, raw honey or maple syrup, sea salt, black pepper, celery seed, and mustard to a large bowl and whisk well.

4 Add the cucumber, cherry tomatoes, dinosaur kale, rinsed black beans, toasted pumpkin seeds, and avocado to the bowl and combine well.

5 Add the cooked quinoa and mix well again so that everything is evenly combined.

6 Serve with optional garnishes, storing any leftovers in the fridge in an airtight container for up to 5 days.

7 Enjoy!

LUNCH

Notes about the recipe: A creamy soup is a wonderful dish to serve or reheat for lunch. Enjoy it just as or with garnishes and a piece of fresh sourdough bread, a side of steamed rice, or over a bowl of creamy polenta.

NUTRITION INFO WITHOUT OPTIONAL GARNISHES:

Calories: 526
Fat: 21g
Carbs: 69g
Net Carbs: 56g
Fiber: 13g
Protein: 19g

Rainbow Veggie Slaw with Baked Tilapia

DAIRY-FREE, GLUTEN-FREE, GRAIN-FREE

The Rainbow Veggie Slaw, with heart-healthy fats from olive oil and tahini, supports hormone health in menopause. Lime adds vitamin C for collagen and immune support while coconut aminos provide amino acids. Almonds offer sleep-promoting magnesium, and the slaw's vegetables deliver antioxidants and fiber for digestive wellness.

For the baked tilapia, simple seasonings and a citrus squeeze yield a lean protein dish, maintaining muscle health, crucial during menopause. This flavorful, nutrient-rich meal is delicious and will help you feel better too.

SERVINGS: 4 • PREP TIME: 20 minutes • COOK TIME: 10 minutes

Baked Tilapia:

- 1 pound (455 g) fresh tilapia filets or 4 medium tilapia filets
- 4 teaspoons (20 ml) olive oil
- 2 teaspoons (12 g) sea salt
- ½ teaspoon (1 g) black pepper
- Squeeze fresh lime or lemon juice

Rainbow Veggie Slaw:

- ¼ cup (60 ml) olive oil
- ¼ cup (60 g) tahini
- 1 tablespoon (15 ml) fresh lime juice
- Zest from ½ medium (0.5 ounces, or 11 g) fresh lime
- 2 tablespoons (28 ml) coconut aminos
- 1 teaspoon (6 g) sea salt
- ½ teaspoon (1 g) black pepper
- 1 tablespoon (10 g) shallot, peeled and minced
- 1 whole medium (0.5 ounces, or 15 g) scallion, minced
- ¼ cup (4 g) minced fresh cilantro, plus 2 tablespoons (2 g) to use as a garnish for the tilapia
- ¼ cup (25 g) chopped almonds
- 4 cups (280 g) shredded green or purple cabbage
- 1 medium (2 ounces, or 60 g) carrot, shredded or julienned
- 1 small (8.5 ounces, or 236 g) green zucchini, shredded, ends removed
- 1 medium (7 ounces, or 196 g) yellow squash, shredded, ends removed

1 Preheat your oven to 400°F (200°C, or gas mark 6).

2 Line a baking tray with parchment paper and place each tilapia filet on the tray. Pat them dry with a paper towel.

3 Spread each tilapia filet with a teaspoon (5 ml) each of olive oil and season with sea salt and black pepper and a squeeze of fresh lime or lemon juice.

4 Bake in the oven until the tilapia flesh is opaque, about 10 minutes.

5 While the tilapia is baking, prepare the Rainbow Veggie Slaw by adding the olive oil, tahini, lime juice, lime zest, coconut aminos, sea salt, and black pepper to a large mixing bowl. Stir together well.

6 Add the shallot, scallion, ¼ cup (4 g) ocilantro, almonds, cabbage, carrot, zucchini, and yellow squash and gently toss until everything is evenly coated in the tahini sauce.

7 When the tilapia is done, remove from the oven. Garnish it with the remaining 2 tablespoons (2 g) cilantro.

8 Serve the Rainbow Veggie Slaw with the Baked Tilapia, storing any leftovers in the fridge in an airtight container. The slaw will keep for 5 days and the tilapia for up to 2 days.

9 Enjoy!

LUNCH

NUTRITION INFO:

Calories: 450
Fat: 32g
Carbs: 15g
Net Carbs: 9g
Fiber: 6g
Protein: 27g

Chicken and Quinoa Immunity Soup with Herbs and Lemon

DAIRY-FREE, GLUTEN-FREE

Quinoa provides complete protein and complex carbohydrates, stabilizing blood sugar levels, which can fluctuate during menopause. Avocado oil, used for cooking chicken or tofu, offers healthy fats beneficial for hormonal balance.

The soup is rich in nutrients. Onions and garlic have natural anti-inflammatory properties, while turmeric, a potent anti-inflammatory agent, may help with joint discomfort common in menopause. Celery and carrots add fiber and essential vitamins.

Fresh ginger can alleviate gastrointestinal discomfort, and coconut milk's healthy fats are good for skin and heart health. The vegetable stock ensures the dish is hydrating, and lemon juice and zest provide a boost of vitamin C.

Nutritional yeast, if used, is a source of B vitamins for energy. Fresh herbs like parsley and basil, along with scallion, add both flavor and additional nutrients beneficial for menopause.

SERVINGS: 4 • PREP TIME: 10 minutes • COOK TIME: 50 minutes

Quinoa:
- 1 cup (173 g) quinoa
- 1 cup (235 ml) low-sodium chicken stock (Replace with vegetable stock to keep this recipe vegetarian and vegan.)
- 1 cup (235 ml) purified water

Chicken:
- 1 tablespoon (15 ml) avocado oil
- 1 pound (455 g) boneless and skinless chicken breast, chopped into bite-sized pieces (Replace with 1 pound [455 g] extra-firm tofu to keep this recipe vegetarian and vegan.)
- 1 teaspoon (6 g) sea salt

Soup:
- 1 medium (5.5 ounces, or 150 g) yellow onion, peeled and minced
- 4 small (1 ounce, or 16 g) garlic cloves, peeled and minced
- 1 teaspoon (6 g) sea salt
- ½ teaspoon (1 g) black pepper
- 1 teaspoon (2 g) celery seed
- 2 teaspoons (4 g) ground turmeric
- 1 cup (100 g) chopped celery, ends removed
- 1 cup (130 g) peeled and chopped carrots, ends removed
- 2 teaspoons (4 g) peeled and minced fresh ginger
- 1 can (14 ounces, or 390 ml) full-fat coconut milk
- 3 cups (700 ml) chicken stock (Use vegetable stock to keep this recipe vegetarian and vegan.)
- 2 bay leaves
- 1 tablespoon (15 ml) fresh lemon juice
- Zest from ½ medium (0.5 ounces, or 13 g) fresh lemon
- 2 tablespoons (8 g) nutritional yeast (optional)

For Garnish:
- ¼ cup (15 g) minced fresh parsley
- 2 tablespoons (6 g) minced fresh basil
- 1 whole medium (0.5 ounces, or 15 g) scallion, minced

1 In a medium saucepan, combine the quinoa, stock, and water. Bring to a boil, reduce the heat to low, cover, and let it simmer for 15 to 20 minutes or until the quinoa is cooked and the liquid is absorbed.

2 While the quinoa is cooking, prepare the chicken or tofu (if preparing the Vegetarian and Vegan option).

3 Add the avocado oil to a large pot and set to medium-low heat. Add the chicken or tofu and season with sea salt. Sauté until cooked through and slightly golden, about 10 minutes. When done, remove from the pot and set aside.

4 Add the onion and garlic to the same pot and season with sea salt, black pepper, celery seed, and turmeric.

5 Sauté until the onions and garlic are soft and a bit golden, 5 to 7 minutes.

6 Add the celery and carrot and continue to sauté until soft, about 5 minutes.

7 Add the ginger and stir very well.

8 Add the canned coconut milk, chicken (or vegetable) stock, and bay leaves. Stir well.

9 Simmer for about 10 minutes.

10 Stir in the cooked chicken (or tofu).

11 Add the lemon juice, lemon zest, and optional nutritional yeast and stir well.

12 When the quinoa is done, remove from the heat, add to the soup, and stir together well. Remove the bay leaves.

13 Serve, garnishing with parsley, basil, and scallion, storing any leftovers in the fridge in an airtight container for up to 3 days.

14 Enjoy!

LUNCH

NUTRITION INFO USING CHICKEN:

Calories: 606
Fat: 30g
Carbs: 40g
Net Carbs: 32g
Fiber: 6g
Protein: 39g

NUTRITION INFO USING TOFU:

Calories: 610
Fat: 33g
Carbs: 42g
Net Carbs: 36g
Fiber: 6g
Protein: 31g

Tofu Stir-Fry with Celery and Bean Sprouts

DAIRY-FREE, GLUTEN-FREE, HIGH-FIBER, HIGH-PROTEIN, VEGETARIAN

Sesame seed oil and coconut aminos offer anti-inflammatory benefits, while rice vinegar aids digestion. Honey and maple syrup provide antioxidants, and black pepper enhances nutrient uptake. Red onions and garlic boost immunity, ginger aids digestion, and tofu supplies phytoestrogens beneficial for menopause. Bean sprouts and celery contribute essential vitamins and fiber, while cashews provide healthy fats and bone-supporting magnesium. Overall, this dish is crafted to address common menopausal concerns.

SERVINGS: 4 • PREP TIME: 15 minutes • COOK TIME: 20 minutes

Sauce:
- 1 tablespoon (15 ml) toasted sesame seed oil
- 2 tablespoons (28 ml) coconut aminos
- 1 tablespoon (15 ml) rice vinegar
- 1 tablespoon (20 g) raw honey or pure maple syrup (Use maple syrup to keep this recipe vegan.)
- ½ teaspoon (1 g) black pepper

Stir-Fry:
- 1 tablespoon (15 ml) toasted sesame seed oil
- 1 medium (5.5 ounces, or 150 g) red onion, peeled and chopped
- 2 small (0.5 ounces, or 8 g) garlic cloves, peeled and minced
- 2 teaspoons (12 g) sea salt
- 1 teaspoon (1 g) dried red pepper flakes
- 1 teaspoon (2 g) peeled and minced fresh ginger
- 2 cups (200 g) chopped celery

- 1 pound (455 g) extra-firm tofu, diced into bite-sized pieces
- 2 cups (208 g) fresh bean sprouts
- 1 whole medium (0.5 ounces, or 15 g) scallion, minced

For Garnish:
- ¼ cup (35 g) chopped cashews

1 Prepare the sauce by whisking the toasted sesame seed oil, coconut aminos, rice vinegar, raw honey or maple syrup, and black pepper in a bowl until it's well combined and creamy. Set aside to use later.

2 In a large sauté pan, add the toasted sesame oil and set the heat to medium-low.

3 Add the red onion and garlic and season with sea salt and red pepper flakes. Sauté the onion until it's soft and translucent, about 5 minutes.

4 Add the ginger and celery and sauté until the celery is tender but still crunchy, about 5 minutes.

5 Add the extra-firm tofu and gently toss and allow it to heat through, tossing often for about 5 minutes.

6 Turn off the heat and gently stir in the sauce, bean sprouts, and scallion.

7 Serve, with chopped cashews, storing any leftovers in the fridge in an airtight container for up to 3 days.

8 Enjoy!

DINNER

Notes about the recipe: Bean sprouts are known to balance your body's cholesterol by reducing your "bad" LDL (low-density lipoprotein) and increasing your "good" HDL (high-density lipoprotein) levels. When you purchase them from your market, be sure to use them within 1 to 2 days, as they do not stay fresh long.

NUTRITION INFO:

Calories: 469
Fat: 29g
Carbs: 37g
Net Carbs: 33g
Fiber: 4g
Protein: 38g

Turkey and Sage-Stuffed Mushrooms with Creamy Polenta

GLUTEN-FREE, HIGH-PROTEIN

This dish is designed to help alleviate menopause symptoms. Vegetable stock and cornmeal offer stable energy, while the dairy-free option avoids hormone-related sensitivities. Portobello mushrooms provide antioxidants that combat age-related oxidative stress. Avocado oil, rich in healthy fats, aids hormone balance. Ground turkey is a lean protein source for muscle maintenance. Onions and garlic support cardiovascular and bone health. Sage may reduce night sweats and hot flashes, while parsley offers anti-inflammatory benefits. Walnuts contribute omega-3s, crucial for cognitive health during menopause.

SERVINGS: 4 • PREP TIME: 10 minutes • COOK TIME: 35 minutes

Creamy Polenta:
- 2 cups (475 ml) vegetable stock
- 1 cup (132 g) fine-grind cornmeal
- ¼ cup (25 g) finely grated Parmesan cheese (Omit to keep this recipe Dairy-Free.)
- 1 teaspoon (6 g) sea salt
- ½ teaspoon (1 g) black pepper

Mushrooms:
- 4 large (340 g) portobello mushrooms, stems removed and wiped clean
- 1 tablespoon (15 ml) avocado oil

Filling:
- 2 tablespoons (28 ml) avocado oil
- 1½ pounds (680 g) ground turkey
- ½ medium (75 g) red onion, peeled and chopped
- 2 small (0.5 ounces, or 8 g) garlic cloves, peeled and minced
- 1 teaspoon (6 g) sea salt
- ½ teaspoon (1 g) black pepper
- 10 fresh sage leaves, minced
- ¼ cup (15 g) minced fresh parsley
- ¼ cup (30 g) chopped walnuts

1 Pour the vegetable stock into a medium sauce-pan and bring to a simmer on the stove over medium heat. Reduce the heat to low and slowly stir in the cornmeal, whisking well so that there are no clumps. Continue to simmer and whisk until the cornmeal is thick and creamy. Stir in the Parmesan cheese, sea salt, and black pepper and set aside the Creamy Polenta to use later.

2 Preheat the oven to 375°F (190°C, or gas mark 5). Brush each mushroom with avocado oil and arrange the mushrooms on a baking tray lined with parchment paper, gill-side up. Bake in the oven for 10 minutes or until they have begun to soften. Remove from the oven and set aside.

3 To prepare the filling, add 1 tablespoon (15 ml) of the avocado oil to a large sauté pan set to medium-low heat.

4 Add the ground turkey and sauté until it's completely cooked though and no longer pink, 5 to 7 minutes, breaking it up with a spatula or wooden spoon as it cooks. When it's done cooking, drain any excess liquids and transfer the turkey to a separate bowl.

5 In the same pan, add the remaining 1 tablespoon (15 ml) of avocado oil, red onion, and garlic and season with sea salt and black pepper. Sauté the onion until it's soft and translucent, about 5 minutes.

6 Add the cooked ground turkey back to the sauté pan and stir well with the red onion and garlic. Add the sage, parsley, and walnuts and stir well so that everything is evenly combined.

7 Fill the mushrooms with the turkey and onion mixture, pressing the filling firmly into each mushroom. Return to the baking sheet and bake for 15 minutes or until the tops begin to crisp and the walnuts have toasted. Remove from the oven and allow to cool for a few minutes before serving.

8 Serve stuffed mushrooms with a side of Creamy Polenta, storing any leftovers in the fridge in an airtight container for up to 3 days.

9 Enjoy!

DINNER

Notes about this recipe: The earthy flavors of sage combine deliciously with portobello mushrooms and turkey. Served with Creamy Polenta, this recipe will surely become one of your favorite healthy meals to prepare!

NUTRITION INFO WITH PARMESAN CHEESE:

Calories: 591
Fat: 30g
Carbs: 39g
Net Carbs: 35g
Fiber: 4g
Protein: 40g

Tempeh and Veggie Skewers

DAIRY-FREE, GLUTEN-FREE, VEGAN, VEGETARIAN

Quinoa is a protein-packed grain that supports muscle health. Including avocado oil and coconut aminos ensures good fats and flavor with reduced sodium. Fresh lime juice and zest not only add citrus flavor but also provide vitamin C. The combination of cumin, black pepper, red pepper flakes, and garlic helps cool inflammation and improve digestion. Tempeh, a fermented soy product, offers phytoestrogens that can help balance hormones. Red onions, bell peppers, mushrooms, and zucchini supply essential vitamins and minerals. The finishing touch of cilantro and scallions adds freshness, while feta provides a calcium boost for bone health.

SERVINGS: 4 • PREP TIME: 10 minutes + 30 minutes to soak wooden skewers • COOK TIME: 20 minutes

Quinoa:
- 1 cup (173 g) quinoa
- 2 cups (475 ml) purified water or low-sodium vegetable stock
- Sea salt to taste (optional)

Skewers:
- 2 tablespoons (28 ml) avocado oil
- 2 tablespoons (28 ml) coconut aminos
- 2 tablespoons (28 ml) fresh lime juice
- Zest from ½ medium (0.5 ounces, or 11 g) fresh lime
- 1 teaspoon (6 g) sea salt
- ½ teaspoon (1 g) black pepper

- 1 teaspoon (2 g) ground cumin
- 1 teaspoon (1 g) dried red pepper flakes
- 2 small (0.5 ounces, or 8 g) garlic cloves, peeled and minced
- 1 pound (455 g) tempeh, cubed
- 1 medium (5.5 ounces, or 150 g) red onion, peeled and cut in 1-inch (2.5 cm) slices
- 1 medium (5.5 ounces, or 150 g) red, orange, or yellow bell pepper, seeded and cut in 1-inch (2.5 cm) strips
- 2 cups (174 g) whole cremini mushrooms, wiped clean
- 2 small (17 ounces, or 472 g) zucchini, ends removed and cut in 1-inch (2.5 cm) rounds

For Garnish:
- ¼ cup (4 g) minced fresh cilantro
- 1 whole medium (0.5 ounces, or 15 g) scallion, minced
- 2 ounces (55 g) crumbled feta cheese (Omit to keep this recipe vegan and dairy-free.)

1 Set aside 8 metal skewers. If using wooden skewers, soak in water for 30 minutes prior to threading.

2 In a medium saucepan, combine the quinoa and water or stock. Bring to a boil, reduce the heat to low, cover, and let it simmer for 15 to 20 minutes or until the quinoa is cooked and the liquid is absorbed. Once it's cooked, fluff it with a fork, cover, and set aside. If preferred, season the quinoa with sea salt to taste.

3 Add the avocado oil, coconut aminos, lime juice, lime zest, sea salt, black pepper, cumin, red pepper flakes, and garlic to a large mixing bowl and whisk well.

4 Add the tempeh and toss well in the marinade.

5 Add the red onion, bell pepper, mushrooms, and zucchini and gently toss until everything is evenly coated in the marinade.

6 Thread each skewer with the tempeh and veggies. Create a pattern threading the tempeh, then each veggie, until you have threaded all the skewers.

7 Heat a grill pan to medium-high. Place each skewer on the pan and allow to sear on each side until the tempeh and veggies are soft and heated through, 3 to 4 minutes per side.

8 Serve and garnish with cilantro, scallion, and a side of quinoa topped with crumbled feta (if using), storing any leftovers in the fridge in an airtight container for up to 3 days.

9 Enjoy!

Notes about this recipe: The skewers are a taste of the veggie rainbow, containing lots of vitamins, minerals, and plenty of plant-based protein from tempeh. These are great to serve at home or to pack on a picnic!

NUTRITION INFO:

Calories: 549
Fat: 20g
Carbs: 75g
Net Carbs: 62g
Fiber: 13g
Protein: 33g

DINNER

Roasted Green Beans and Tofu Over Kale with Spiced Peanut Sauce

DAIRY-FREE, GLUTEN-FREE, GRAIN-FREE, VEGAN, VEGETARIAN

Green beans and tofu offer protein and menopause-relieving isoflavones, vital for aging muscles and hormonal balance. Avocado oil and olive oil contribute heart-healthy fats important for cardiovascular wellness post-menopause. Kale, rich in calcium and vitamins, supports bone health, while nutritional yeast adds energy-boosting B vitamins.

The Peanut Sauce, with apple cider vinegar and garlic, aids digestion and immunity. Sesame seeds and cilantro in the garnish provide essential minerals and detoxifying benefits, creating a nutritious dish that supports your body's defenses during menopause

SERVINGS: 4 • PREP TIME: 10 minutes • COOK TIME: 35 minutes

Green Beans and Tofu:
- 1 pound (456g) green beans, ends removed
- 1 medium (1.5 ounces, or 40 g) shallot
- 1 pound (456 g) extra-firm tofu (Replace with 1 pound [455 g] boneless and skinless chicken breast if desired.)
- 2 tablespoons (28 ml) avocado oil
- 1 teaspoon (6 g) sea salt
- ½ teaspoon (1 g) black pepper

Kale:
- 2 tablespoons (28 ml) avocado oil
- 2 tablespoons (28 ml) fresh lime juice
- ½ teaspoon (3 g) sea salt
- 1 tablespoon (8 g) nutritional yeast
- 8 cups (536 g) chopped dinosaur kale

Peanut Sauce:
- ¼ cup (64 g) natural peanut butter (creamy or crunchy)
- 1 tablespoon (15 ml) olive oil
- 1 tablespoon (15 ml) raw apple cider vinegar
- 1 tablespoon (15 ml) coconut aminos
- 1 small (0.1 ounces, or 4 g) garlic clove, peeled and minced
- 1 teaspoon (6 g) sea salt
- ½ teaspoon (1 g) black pepper
- Purified water (optional)

For Garnish:
- 1 tablespoon (8 g) black or white sesame seeds
- ¼ cup (4 g) minced fresh cilantro

1 Preheat your oven to 425°F (220°C, or gas mark 7).

2 Chop the green beans into bite-sized pieces.

3 Peel the shallot and mince it very small.

4 Pat the tofu dry (or chicken breast if you are preparing the non-vegetarian and non-vegan option) and dice into bite-sized pieces.

5 Add the avocado oil to a large mixing bowl, followed by the sea salt and black pepper.

6 Gently toss the green beans and tofu (or chicken breast) in the avocado oil mixture until everything is coated.

7 Arrange on a baking tray lined with parchment paper and bake in the oven for 30 to 35 minutes, tossing at the halfway mark.

8 While the Green Beans and Tofu (or chicken breast) are baking, prepare the kale. Add the avocado oil to a large mixing bowl, followed by the lime juice, sea salt, and nutritional yeast. Stir together well.

9 Add the chopped dinosaur kale and massage into the mixture until the kale has become softer and fully coated. Set aside.

10 Prepare the Peanut Sauce by adding all the ingredients into a blender and blending on high until very creamy, scraping down the sides of the blender as needed. If it's too thick for your preference, add 1 tablespoon (15 ml) water and blend again, repeating until it's to your liking. Pour into a glass jar until ready to serve.

11 Remove the Green Beans and Tofu (or chicken) from the oven and toss with the massaged kale. Serve with the Peanut Sauce, and garnish with black or white sesame seeds and cilantro, storing any leftovers in the fridge in an airtight container for up to 5 days.

12 Enjoy!

DINNER

NUTRITION INFO:

Calories: 590
Fat: 35g
Carbs: 36g
Net Carbs: 30g
Fiber: 6g
Protein: 31g

Farro and Black Bean One-Pot Wonder

HIGH-FIBER, VEGETARIAN

Greek yogurt in the Lime-Zested Yogurt Sauce offers calcium for bone health, while lime provides vitamin C for immune support. Avocado oil in the Farro and Black Beans adds heart-healthy fats, and the aromatic garlic and onion help with hormone balance. Spices like cumin and paprika support digestion, and tomato products contribute lycopene for heart health.

Farro, or gluten-free brown rice, and black beans supply fiber and protein, essential for muscle and digestive health during menopause. Baby spinach adds iron, and the dish is topped with Lime-Zested Yogurt and cilantro for extra flavor and nutrients, supporting overall fitness in menopause.

SERVINGS: 4 • PREP TIME: 10 minutes • COOK TIME: 30–45 minutes

Lime-Zested Yogurt Sauce:
- 1 cup (227 g) 2% plain Greek yogurt (Use dairy-free plain yogurt to keep this recipe.)
- 1 tablespoon (15 ml) fresh lime juice
- Zest from 1 medium (0.5 ounces, or 11 g) fresh lime
- Pinch fine sea salt
- Black pepper to taste

Farro and Black Beans:
- 2 tablespoons (28 ml) avocado oil
- ½ medium (75 g) red onion, peeled and diced
- 3 small (0.5 ounces, or 12 g) garlic cloves, peeled and minced
- 1 teaspoon (6 g) sea salt
- ½ teaspoon (1 g) black pepper
- 1 teaspoon (2 g) ground cumin
- 1 teaspoon (2 g) smoked paprika
- ½ teaspoon (1 g) ground cardamom
- 6 ounces (170 g) tomato paste
- 1 cup (208 g) pearled farro (Use brown rice to keep this recipe gluten free.)

- 15 ounces (425 g) cooked black beans, rinsed
- 1 can (28 ounces, or 795 g) fire-roasted diced tomatoes
- 1 cup (235 ml) vegetable stock
- 4 cups (172 g) chopped baby spinach (or another leafy green)

For Garnish:
- ½ cup (8 g) minced fresh cilantro

1 Prepare the Lime-Zested Yogurt Sauce by mixing the Greek yogurt (or dairy-free yogurt) in a bowl with the lime juice and zest, sea salt, and black pepper. Set aside to use later.

2 Add the avocado oil to a large Dutch oven or stockpot and set to medium-low heat.

3 Add the red onion and garlic and sauté until the red onion has softened, about 5 minutes.

4 Season with sea salt, black pepper, cumin, smoked paprika, and cardamom and stir well.

5 Add the tomato paste and stir very well.

6 Add the pearled farro (or brown rice), black beans, fire-roasted tomatoes, and vegetable stock and bring to a boil.

7 Once boiling, reduce the heat to a simmer and cover the pot with it slightly vented, for about 15 minutes (if using farro) or about 30 minutes (if using brown rice). Stir a few times while cooking. The farro (or brown rice) will be done when it absorbs most of the pot's liquids and is very soft. Taste-test if you are not sure.

8 Turn off the heat and stir in the baby spinach (or leafy green of choice). Let it wilt in the pot.

9 Serve topped with the Lime-Zested Yogurt Sauce and garnished with cilantro, storing any leftovers in the fridge in an airtight container for up to 5 days.

10 Enjoy!

DINNER

NUTRITION INFO:

Calories: 465
Fat: 9g
Carbs: 71g
Net Carbs: 0g
Fiber: 11g
Protein: 23g

Beef and Blueberry Walnut Stir-Fry Over Wild Rice

DAIRY-FREE, GLUTEN-FREE, HIGH-FIBER, HIGH-PROTEIN

Toasted walnuts and ground beef in the stir-fry provide essential omega-3s and protein for heart and muscle health during menopause. Sea salt and herbs like fennel seeds support digestion, while blueberries and spinach offer antioxidants and nutrients for bone health. Parsley and sage can help with hormonal balance. Wild rice is a fiber-rich carbohydrate, good for energy levels and blood sugar management during menopause.

SERVINGS: 4 • PREP TIME: 15 minutes • COOK TIME: 20–30 minutes

Wild Rice:
- 1½ cups (240 g) wild rice
- 3 cups (700 ml) purified water

Stir-Fry:
- ½ cup (60 g) chopped raw walnuts
- 1 pound (455 g) ground beef
- 2 teaspoons (12 g) sea salt
- 1 teaspoon (2 g) black pepper
- 2 teaspoons (4 g) dried fennel seeds
- 1 cup (145 g) fresh blueberries
- 4 cups (172 g) baby spinach, chopped
- ¼ cup (15 g) minced fresh parsley
- 5–6 fresh sage leaves, minced

1 Prepare the wild rice by adding the wild rice and water to a saucepan and set the stove's heat to medium-high. When the rice begins to boil, reduce the heat to low and cover the pan with a lid, slightly vented. Simmer for 20 to 30 minutes until the rice absorbs all the water and is light and fluffy.

2 To toast the walnuts, preheat your oven to 350°F (180°C, or gas mark 4). Spread the walnuts evenly on a baking tray lined with parchment paper. Bake in the oven until the walnuts are golden in color and become fragrant, 5 to 7 minutes. Keep an eye on them so that they don't burn. Remove from the oven and transfer to a bowl to cool.

3 Add the ground beef to a large pot and set the heat to medium-low. Sauté until it's completely cooked though and no longer pink, 5 to 7 minutes, breaking it up with a spatula or wooden spoon as it cooks.

4 Season the beef with sea salt, black pepper, and fennel seeds and stir well.

5 When it's done cooking, turn off the heat and drain any excess liquids.

6 Add the blueberries, baby spinach, parsley, sage, and toasted walnuts and stir well together.

7 Serve with the Wild Rice, storing any leftovers in the fridge in an airtight container for up to 3 days.

8 Enjoy!

DINNER

NUTRITION INFO:

Calories: 581
Fat: 29g
Carbs: 53g
Net Carbs: 47g
Fiber: 6g
Protein: 30g

Seasoned Lamb with Roasted Golden Veggies

DAIRY-FREE, GLUTEN-FREE, HIGH-FIBER, HIGH-PROTEIN

Avocado oil provides healthy fats for hormonal health in menopause, while red onion and garlic boast anti-oxidants to keep you strong. Sea salt and black pepper are essential minerals, and red pepper flakes can offer a metabolism boost. Oregano and fennel seeds help with digestion and sage with cognitive function, both areas affected by menopause. Ground lamb is a rich protein source, with a tofu alternative for those prefer-ring plant-based options.

The veggies, including butternut squash, beets, and carrots, are packed with vitamins, fiber, and beta-carotene, supporting immune function and skin health, which can decline during menopause. Fresh herbs like cilantro and parsley have detoxifying properties and add a flavor boost, making this dish a delightful, nutrient-dense option for menopausal dietary needs.

SERVINGS: 4 • PREP TIME: 15 minutes • COOK TIME: 30 minutes

Veggies:
- 2 cups (340 g) peeled and cubed butternut squash
- 1 cup (136 g) peeled and chopped golden beets
- 2 medium (4 ounces, or 120 g) carrots, chopped
- 2 tablespoons (28 ml) avocado oil
- 1 teaspoon (6 g) sea salt
- ½ teaspoon (1 g) black pepper

Lamb:
- 1 tablespoon (15 ml) avocado oil
- ½ medium (75 g) red onion, peeled and chopped
- 2 small (0.5 ounces, or 8 g) garlic cloves, peeled and minced
- 2 teaspoons (12 g) sea salt
- ½ teaspoon (1 g) black pepper
- 1 teaspoon (1 g) dried red pepper flakes

- 2 teaspoons (2 g) dried oregano
- 2 teaspoons (4 g) dried fennel seeds
- 5–7 fresh sage leaves, minced
- 1 pound (455 g) ground lamb (Replace with 1 pound [455 g] extra-firm tofu to keep this recipe vegan and vegetarian.)
- ¼ cup (4 g) minced fresh cilantro or (15 g) fresh parsley

1 Preheat the oven to 400°F (200°C, or gas mark 6).

2 Line a baking tray with parchment paper. Toss the butternut squash, golden beets, and carrots with the avocado oil, sea salt, and black pepper in a large bowl until the veggies are coated in the oil and seasonings.

3 Spread the veggies on the baking tray and roast in the oven until soft and slightly caramelized, about 30 minutes, tossing after 15 minutes.

4 While the veggies are roasting, prepare the lamb mixture.

5 In a large sauté pan, add the avocado oil and set the heat to medium-low.

6 Add the red onion and garlic, and season with sea salt, black pepper, red pepper flakes, oregano, fennel seeds, and sage. Sauté the onion until it's soft and translucent, about 5 minutes.

7 Add the ground lamb and sauté until it's completely cooked though and no longer pink, about 10 minutes, breaking it up with a spatula or wooden spoon. If using tofu, break it up with your hands as you add it to the pan. Stir it often until it heats through, about 5 minutes.

8 Turn off the heat and stir in the roasted butternut, golden beets, and carrots.

9 Stir in the freshly minced cilantro or parsley.

10 Serve, storing any leftovers in the fridge in an airtight container for up to 3 days.

11 Enjoy!

DINNER

Notes about the recipe: Serve this with a side of brown rice or quinoa, for additional healthy carbs and fiber.

NUTRITION INFO USING LAMB:

Calories: 487
Fat: 37g
Carbs: 18g
Net Carbs: 13g
Fiber: 5g
Protein: 21g

NUTRITION INFO USINGTOFU:

Calories: 303
Fat: 18g
Carbs: 19g
Net Carbs: 14g
Fiber: 5g
Protein: 19g

Pistachio Matcha Bliss Balls

DAIRY-FREE, GLUTEN-FREE, GRAIN-FREE, VEGAN, VEGETARIAN

Dried dates and matcha powder provide a sustained energy boost, beneficial during menopause. Pistachios and pine nuts offer healthy fats for hormonal support, while sea salt helps maintain electrolyte balance. Vanilla bean powder can help soothe mood swings, and coconut oil with shredded coconut delivers medium-chain triglycerides and fiber for weight and digestive health. This combination makes for a welcoming menopause snack that's both nutritious and satisfying.

SERVINGS: 12 • PREP TIME: 10 minutes • COOK TIME: 0 minutes

- 1 cup (225 g) whole dried dates, pitted and chopped
- 1 cup (123 g) raw pistachios
- ½ cup (68 g) raw pine nuts
- Pinch sea salt
- 1 teaspoon (4 g) vanilla bean powder
- 2 teaspoons (4 g) culinary-grade matcha
- 1 tablespoon (14 g) coconut oil, melted
- 1 ounce (28 g) dried and unsweetened shredded coconut

1 Cover the dates with hot water and let sit for 10 minutes.

2 While the dates are soaking, pulse the pistachios and pine nuts in a food processor until fine and crumbly. Add in the sea salt, vanilla bean powder, matcha, and coconut oil and pulse until well combined.

3 Drain the dates and add to the food processor, pulsing until everything is well combined and a "dough" has formed.

4 Using 1 tablespoon (15 g) measuring spoon, scoop a spoonful of the dough and roll into a ball with your hands. Continue until you have used all the dough (about 12 balls).

5 Roll each ball in the shredded coconut.

6 Serve, storing any leftovers in the fridge in an airtight container for up to 2 weeks or in the freezer for up to 3 months.

7 Enjoy!

NUTRITION INFO:

Calories: 157
Fat: 9g
Carbs: 19g
Net Carbs: 16g
Fiber: 3g
Protein: 3g

Raw Avocado Key Lime Pie

DAIRY-FREE, GLUTEN-FREE, GRAIN-FREE, VEGAN, VEGETARIAN

Walnuts and macadamia nuts provide healthy fats and protein, supporting hormonal balance and heart health, key concerns during menopause. Unsweetened coconut and dates contain fiber and add natural sweetness without spiking blood sugar. The avocado filling is rich in monounsaturated fats, which are crucial for skin health and to maintain healthy cholesterol levels.

SERVINGS: 8 • PREP TIME: 20 minutes • COOK TIME: 0 minutes + 4 hours to freeze

Crust:
- 1 cup (100 g) raw walnuts
- 1 cup (125 g) raw macadamia nuts
- ¾ cup (60 g) shredded, dried, and unsweetened coconut
- 1½ cups (338 g) whole dried dates, pitted
- 1 teaspoon (5 ml) pure vanilla extract
- Pinch sea salt

Filling:
- 4 medium (600 g) avocados, peeled and pitted
- ½ cup (120 ml) fresh lime juice
- 2 tablespoons (12 g) fresh lime zest
- ¼ cup (80 g) pure maple syrup
- 2 teaspoons (9 g) vanilla bean powder OR 1 teaspoon (5 ml) pure vanilla extract

For Garnish (Optional):
- ¼ cup (36 g) fresh blueberries
- 2 tablespoons (10 g) shredded, dried, and unsweetened coconut
- Fresh lime slices
- Fresh mint leaves

1 Pulse the crust ingredients in a food processor until fine and crumbly, scraping down the sides of the bowl as needed. Using your hands, press firmly, creating a crust into an 8-inch (20-cm) tart pan lined with parchment paper. Be sure to press the crust up the sides of the pan.

2 Prepare the filling by adding all the filling ingredients to a high-speed blender and pulsing until very creamy. Pour the key lime filling into the crust and spread it evenly with the back of a spoon or baker's spatula. Transfer to the freezer and completely freeze (about 4 hours or overnight).

3 Remove from the freezer before serving and if desired, garnish with the optional blueberries, dried coconut, lime slices, and mint leaves.

4 Serve, storing any leftovers in the fridge in an airtight container for up to 5 days.

5 Enjoy!

NUTRITION INFO WITHOUT GARNISH:

Calories: 472
Fat: 34g
Carbs: 44g
Net Carbs: 32g
Fiber: 12g
Protein: 8g

NUTRITION INFO WITH GARNISH:

Calories: 483
Fat: 34g
Carbs: 45g
Net Carbs: 33g
Fiber: 12g
Protein: 8g

DESSERTS/TREATS

Acknowledgments

Never in a million years did I ever believe that I would have the opportunity to write a book. So, when I got the chance, I was extremely cautious, Iand wondered, "Can I do this?"

A big thank-you goes to my dad, who always said to me as a child, "There is no such word as can't." With that advice, I grabbed the opportunity with both hands and poured my heart and soul into every page. Thank you to my wonderful mum for her words of wisdom from the very beginning when I would share my first drafts to her and received the constructive criticism I so needed. The love and encouragement from both of you has always been there driving me forward.

Sam, where would I be without your morning voice notes? Full of enthusiasm and positivity, you were the person to lift me up on the days I found it tough to keep writing.

Christina, you told me I was perimenopausal when I didn't want to hear it. You also said everything would be okay because I wasn't going crazy. I just want to say thank you for inspiring me every day and cheering me on.

Jill Alexander, my editor, your faith in me and your passionate support for this project have been nothing short of transformative. Your guidance has been a shining light, instilling in me the confidence that my thoughts could be translated into this book.

Chrystle Fiedler, my developmental editor, your words of encouragement and praise meant more to me than I think you will ever know. Your magic touch to the book has helped everything come together before my eyes. I can't thank you enough.

Larry, my husband, your unwavering support has been my rock. You've understood my absences as I poured myself into writing. Now, as I return to our shared evenings, perhaps we can find something we both enjoy on TV—something other than football!

To the Cara Fitness community, without you, this book would remain unwritten. Your stories, loyalty, and unwavering support, especially during my recovery from spinal surgery, have taught me the infinite value of shared narratives. We each have a story, none greater than the next, for we are all unique and special. My love for our fitness family knows no bounds.

Finally, my girls, Sian and Danielle. The two most beautiful humans in the world. Life hasn't always been easy for you growing up with a mother that didn't always make the best life decisions. Despite the crazy childhood, you have both grown up to be women that I am so proud of. The biggest thank-you goes to you both for always believing in me, driving me forward, and wanting me to be the best that I could be for you. I love you to the moon and back.

Thank you to you all!

About Cara Metz

Cara Metz is not just an advocate for women's fitness; she is a living testament to the transformative power of healthy living. As a former Open British Latin American Dance Champion, Cara's journey in the world of health and fitness began on the dance floor, gracing international stages as a competitor, teacher, and coach. However, it was her personal battle with burnout and an eating disorder that ignited her commitment to wellness.

Retiring from professional dancing in 1996, Cara channelled her energy into fitness instruction. By 2002, she had expanded her expertise to personal training. Her own experiences with perimenopause propelled her to become a certified MenoFit™ instructor, deepening her knowledge in menopause fitness and nutrition.

The Cara Fitness app, born from her desire to support and empower, has become a digital sanctuary for thousands of women seeking guidance and transformation. The app's philosophy is simple yet powerful: Fitness should be accessible, achievable, and adaptable, even with just fifteen minutes a day.

Beyond the app, Cara is a dynamic motivational speaker and an authoritative voice in menopause fitness. She regularly engages her substantial social media following and the Cara Fitness community through online workshops, sharing insights and inspiration.

Cara's career is dedicated to uplifting women at a stage often overlooked by the fitness industry. Her approach is both a beacon of hope and a blueprint for aging gracefully, energetically, and with vitality. Through Cara Fitness, she is not just changing routines—she is changing lives.

Resources

Useful Websites and Communities

- **Menopause Support:** menopausesupport.co.uk
- **The North American Menopause Society:** menopause.org
- **Dr. Mary Claire Haver:** galvestondiet.com
- **The British Menopause Society (BMS):** thebms.org.uk
- **Cara Fitness:** carafitness.co.uk

Midlife Podcasts

- The Dr. Louise Newson Podcast
- The Happy Menopause
- Listen Up MIDLIFE CONVERSATIONS

Menopause Books

- *The Happy Menopause* by Jackie Lynch
- *Menopausing* by Davina McCall
- *The Galveston Diet* by Dr. Mary Claire Haver
- *The New Menopause* by Dr. Mary Claire Haver
- *The Definitive Guide to Perimenopause and Menopause* by Dr. Louise Newson
- *Next Level* by Dr. Stacy T. Sims

Apps

- Cara Fitness
- Balance
- ZenMe
- Unplug
- Insight Timer

Index